Psychology Discourse Practice

Psychology Discourse Practice:
From Regulation to Resistance

**Erica Burman, Gill Aitken,
Pam Alldred, Robin Allwood,
Tom Billington, Brenda Goldberg,
Ángel Gordo López, Colleen Heenan,
Deb Marks and Sam Warner**

UNIVERSITY OF WOLVERHAMPTON
LIBRARY
F312
Acc No. 2105017
CLASS 150.
CONTROL 0748405038
DATE 20. AUG 1997
SITE WV
PSY
WITHDRAWN

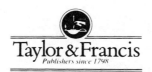
Taylor & Francis
Publishers since 1798

UK	Taylor & Francis Ltd, 1 Gunpowder Square, London EC4A 3DE
USA	Taylor & Francis Inc., 1900 Frost Road, Suite 101, Bristol, PA 19007

© Erica Burman, Gill Aitken, Pam Alldred, Robin Allwood, Tom Billington, Brenda Goldberg, Ángel Gordo López, Colleen Heenan, Deb Marks and Sam Warner, 1996

*All rights reserved. No part of this publication may be repro-
duced, stored in a retrieval system, or transmitted, in any form
or by any means, electronic, mechanical, photocopying,
recording or otherwise, without the prior permission of the
Publisher.*

First published 1996

**A Catalogue Record for this book is available from the British
Library**

ISBN 0 7484 0503 8
ISBN 0 7484 0504 6 (pbk)

**Library of Congress Cataloging-in-Publication Data are
available on request**

Typeset in 10/12 pt Times
by Best-set Typesetter Ltd, Hong Kong

Printed by SRP Ltd, Exeter

Contents

Contents

Acknowledgments and permissions

Specific acknowledgments accompany individual chapters. However, in addition to these, the authors would like to gratefully acknowledge the support of the Discourse Unit at the Department of Psychology and Speech Pathology, the Manchester Metropolitan University, whose existence made possible, and provided a frame for, this book – at least for some of us; the psychology technicians for their patient help throughout, especially at the end; and Brenda for the last-minute compiling. Anwar Hussain and Harvey Budworth were unable to see this project through to completion, but we would like to acknowledge their contributions in its early stages.

For permission to reproduce materials, we acknowledge the British Psychological Society (for Table 5.1 in Chapter 5); the Museum of London (for the illustrations in Chapter 9) and Mapleleaf Holdings (for the illustrations in Chapter 10).

The Authors
November 1995

Chapter 1

Psychology discourse practice: From regulation to resistance

Erica Burman

Like every other book, this volume tells a story. This book is about the role psychological knowledge and practices play in shaping and governing our lives. We address how psychology functions within current institutionalized structures of inequality. Our account is for people engaged with the practice or the theory of psychology – whether as professional psychologists, or as health and welfare professionals drawing on psychological concepts and methods in their work, or as undergraduate and postgraduate students in search of a more reflexive and institutionally located analysis of the discipline. This is a polemical as well as a pedagogical story, in that we seek to engage and persuade as well as inform. Like the readers we address, our writing spans the range of applications of psychology, as theory and as practice, in the senses not only of explicit professional expertise and activity but also as an implicit ingredient in our everyday lives. We explore how we as the authors, like you, the readers, are multiply positioned in relation to psychology and the material in this book. We treat this diversity of background and stance as an important resource and topic, both for the contents and the uses of this book.

This chapter, therefore, serves to outline the key concepts and questions that structure this volume. We aim to show how psychology functions within contemporary Western societies, informing education, health and welfare practices as well as theory and social policy. Focusing on particular practical arenas, we show how psychological effects are more than discursive in that they enter into the material structure of the major institutions that govern our experience as well as our actions. However, while our story does not guarantee a happy ending, it is not entirely gloomy either. The subtitle of this book, 'from regulation to resistance', reflects our concern to go beyond the determinism of structures and resignation to the ways these oppress and regulate us, to elaborate strategies and document activities that – in theoretical, methodological, professional and everyday arenas – offer some scope for movement and change. In this sense, this book is rooted in very practical concerns and we hope it will help to support some very practical interventions. But now for some clarification of our framework.

Erica Burman

Psychology as a practice

In this book we start from the position that psychology is not merely a body of theory that lies in textbooks, but informs the ways we live and understand our experiences. Who 'we' are and how generally we can lay claim to a common set of experiences or practices, either as authors or as social subjects generally, is a theme addressed in each chapter. It also connects closely with the crucial political questions about action. But what brings us together to write this book, and interpellates you to read it, is how psychological ideas both inform and reflect the modern industrialized context that gave rise to them. The standards by which we evaluate normality and abnormality, social adjustment, mental illness or disability, are all informed by theories and technologies of assessment and testing. While these reflect particular values and orientations, they work to scientize and naturalize the particularity and partiality of their perspectives.

But we would be overstating the influence of psychology and our responsibilities for its effects if we imagined that psychology does this alone. For psychologists are not the only ones to mobilize and dispense this knowledge. Psychiatrists, social workers, nurses, teachers, health visitors and community workers employ these ideas in their work and indeed in some cases their professions are structured around particular psychological theories such as the role of early experience in later social or personal disturbance. Our experience in the twentieth-century Western world is correspondingly organized according to the 'psychological complex' (Ingleby, 1985; Rose, 1985) characterized by the proliferation of psychological discourses which construct us as individuals with rights, responsibilities and stably constituted proclivities and attributes.

Thus in this book we discuss how the domain of psychological expertise extends from the evaluation of the home, family forms and childrearing practices (see Chapters 7 and 8), to school (Chapter 3), from the psychiatric (Chapters 4, 5, 6 and 10) to the legal (Chapters 3 and 5). Psychological theories are invoked in relation to the most external and naked structuring of constraints on our lives, as in removing children from families (Chapter 8), or incarceration in special hospitals (Chapter 5), to the most apparently intimate and spontaneous features of our experience, such as gender, humour (Chapter 9) and sexuality (Chapter 10).

In attending to the role of psychology within social practices, therefore, we are referring to the domains of application in which psychological knowledge is used to legitimize actions and interventions. This moves us beyond the scrutiny of particular arenas of professional practice (although we also deal with their specificities), to explore the more generalized effects of psychological theories and techniques. We are concerned with what the feminist sociologist Dorothy Smith (1990) calls 'the relations of ruling', in which psychological technologies (in the form of theoretical edifices or testing devices, as well as specific professional agents) play an important role.

In this book we address the ways psychology affects, intersects with and (re)constitutes inequalities structured around gender, 'race', class, age, sexuality and disability. This is not to say that psychology is exclusively responsible for these oppressions and inequalities, but that it currently collaborates in maintaining them. This collusion is explicitly structured into its practices, as where professional psychologists, as gatekeepers to specialist institutions and services, police the boundaries between normality and abnormality. It also functions implicitly in the ways psychological ideas inform our ways of experiencing our lives through its seepage into, and reflection of, popular cultural forms. As already indicated, the purpose of this book is not only to pose questions about the practices we inhabit and perform, but to identify ways of intervening in these so that we can change them. This is a project which engages not only students and practitioners of psychology, but all of us who as professionals or as individuals subscribe to psychological notions about ourselves and our relationships as part of contemporary cultural life.

How to read this book

The book is divided into three sections. These are organized according to the stance and progression of ideas rather than topic. Part I, Instituting agencies, addresses the forms of experience produced through institutional practices, to consider how – as practitioners, laypeople and theorists – we collude with, or can counter, the institutionally constructed positions we occupy. The chapters in this part address these themes through a focus on self-help texts on depression (in Chapter 2), on educational psychological assessments and interventions (Chapter 3) and the contested and contradictory project of 'feminist therapy'. Here the disjunction between institutional location and more local discursive positionings emerges as an important resource and, in Chapter 4, this is explicitly addressed in terms of the opportunities afforded by a discourse analytic approach in reflecting on therapeutic practice. Despite their diverse topics and frameworks, these chapters share a common focus on the political ambiguities of expertise and interpretation; the role of institutional power relations in the creation of forms of subjectivity.

Part II, 'Practicing (at) the limits of representation', deals more specifically with the (legal, psychiatric and research) processes by which certain groups (children, 'dangerous' women, black women) suffer further stigmatization through their failure to conform to normalized categories. The notion of 'representation' used here does not allude to a cognitive, individual perceptual function, nor to the political process of democratic participation through delegation, but to a cultural practice according to which certain experiences or identities are systematically disallowed and – in some cases literally – contained or excluded. Clinical and educational psychologists help to demarcate domains of (in Chapters 5 and 6) femininity (in Chapter 5 addressing the racialization of femininity) and (in Chapter 7) childhood. But these chapters do not make the corresponding error of romanticizing the positions of subordination/exclusion to treat these as authentic repositories of alternative perspectives. Rather the focus is on how current dominant representational practices systematically reproduce those experiences that lie outside their limits. Moreover, those so positioned are not passive but can comment on these processes.

Part III, 'Dis/locating institutional boundaries', develops the theme of negotiation of multiple positions and the scope this offers for intervention in relation to practical, everyday and theoretical arenas. The focus here is on how the contradictory positionings can form a resource for the elaboration of resistance to institutional definitions and categorizations, with the topics covered ranging from evaluation of mothering (Chapter 8), to commentary and cultural intervention with an analysis of the ways women use and are abused by humour (Chapter 9), to the more apparently material cultural categorizations performed by gender identity clinics (Chapter 10).

The structure of this book therefore traces the development of perspective and argument rather than a compartmentalization according to arena. We have avoided the conventional divisions between theory and practice, between clinical and educational arenas, between method and application. These polarities themselves reinscribe hierarchies within the discipline of psychology, and function to separate conceptual and practical work according to a very traditional (and traditionally gendered) division of labour. This book therefore attempts to disrupt these institutional power relations and, as illustrated by its organization, to afford other ways of coordinating the interests and activities that enjoin us in writing and reading this work. However, by focusing on some areas more than others you may wish to trace another equally viable route through this book. In the rest of this chapter we highlight some of the presuppositions underlying this book, in which we also identify non-chronologically organized themes that may guide reading trajectories.

Discourse and psychology

The concept of discourse has acquired a wide currency in academic discussions across the social sciences, literary theory and philosophy. We use it here to connect with debates about the role and functions of psychology, taking psychology in its broadest senses as outlined above. Ideas about discourse have entered psychology over the last decade in the form of discussions about the importance of language in constructing our understandings of the world we live in. The 'crisis' in psychology of the 1970s reflected an increasing disenchantment with psychology's models and methods. Mainstream psychology investigated its subject matter – people – as isolated individuals, rather than as members of specific social and cultural practices. This impoverished view was made possible by psychology's failure to theorize language. The world was treated as a silent place (Parker, 1989). Psychology has failed to address the way discourses mark out positions for us as individuals within liberal democracies. Moreover, psychology has failed to reflect on its own culturally privileged (white, male, Western, ruling class, heterosexual, able-bodied . . .) position. In these ways psychological theory has severed individuals from social and institutional practices. Socially produced characteristics and relationships are treated as properties of individuals. Thus individuals can be treated as the originators of, or responsible for, the circumstances that they suffer. This accounts for the role of psychology in pathologizing those who fail to fit its norms.

The 'crisis' in psychology of the 1960s and 1970s was primarily concerned with questioning the ethics and applicability of psychological research methods (Harré and Secord, 1972). Traditional positivist approaches treated people as 'subjects' to be manipulated, and to be theorized about in terms of scientific laws of cause and effect (e.g. Reason and Rowan, 1981). The 'new paradigm' approaches emerging from 'the crisis' criticized such mechanistic models which ignored human agency and meaning-making activities, and excluded questions of power by excising the researcher's role in the name of hygienic, objective research. Instead, the 'new paradigm' approach aimed to democratize research practices through recognizing the humanity of psychological subjects (of the researchers as well as the researched) and theorizing both research processes and psychological theory as constructed by negotiated realities.

But while positivist psychology observed people and new paradigm research addressed the involvement of the researcher, discourse work makes a further qualitative shift to locate psychology within the social structures that produced and maintain it as a discipline and which it in turn produces and maintains. While new paradigm work attempts to construct a (more) authentic account of experience, to correct the dehumanization of previous research practices, the turn to deconstruction puts the category of experience itself into question. Acccording to discourse approaches all knowledge – including, and perhaps especially, self-knowledge – is socially constituted.

In terms of the status of psychological knowledge, a key consequence is that disciplinary boundaries no longer hold in rigid or distinct ways, so that we might perhaps engage in literary or cultural analysis to inform our discursive analyses. Moreover, this attention to the cultural sources of subjectivity enables a critical perspective on psychology as fundamentally and intrinsically individualizing. If positivist psychology unreflexively takes the individual as its research object (and robs it of its subjectivity), then new paradigm work attempts to restore this subjectivity and treat experience as a research resource. The further conceptual move made by discourse and deconstructionist approaches is to take experience itself as an effect, as constructed by and through institutional practices, in which psychology plays a key role.

The variety of discourse analysis that we subscribe to here is concerned with the social construction and constitution of the categories of experience, or subjectivities. While some chapters explicitly discuss the significance of particular linguistic formulations, this is to explore the positions and identities these set up, rather than an exposition of linguistic rules and roles. Discourse is therefore understood as both institutional medium *and* practice, as both producing and enacting institutional relations. In this we draw on other accounts that apply post-structuralist and social constructionist ideas to psychology such as Henriques *et al.* (1984); Rose (1985, 1989); Billig *et al.* (1988); Walkerdine (1988); Hollway (1989); Parker and Shotter (1990); Parker (1992); Burman and Parker (1993); Curt (1994); Burman (1994a). While some of these accounts are concerned with specific arenas of psychological practice (e.g. Rose, 1985, 1989; Walkerdine, 1988; and Burman, 1994a with developmental psychology; Parker, 1992 with social psychology, or Hollway, 1989, with 'methods'), others put forward a more wide-ranging account of the functioning of psychology (Henriques *et al.*, 1984; Parker and Shotter, 1990; Parker *et al.*, 1995). This book connects those critiques of the discipline of academic psychology with others focusing on its clinical and educational arenas of practice (e.g. Banton *et al.*, 1985; Pilgrim and Treacher, 1991; Boyle, 1992).

Using a Foucauldian approach, Parker (1992, p. 5) defines discourse as 'a system of statements that constructs an object'. In this book we explore the consequences of the categories and relations elaborated within psychological discourses and the ways they intersect with other institutional practices. We ask how certain categories have been produced and constituted as topics and what issues and relations this conceptual landscape highlights or occludes. For example, analysing the positions of Asian and African Caribbean women, Chapter 5 illustrates how the policy focus on black men in mental health services articulates both the invisibility of gender in debates on 'race' and the failure to theorize 'race' and cultural differences adequately within feminist theories. This conceptual silence is reflected as a significant absence in mental health services, both at the level of policy and practice. Similarly, Chapter 6 addresses the agencies and responsibilities made possible by portraying women who have been sexually abused as either 'victims' or 'survivors', in relation to the identities mapped out for the women, the provision of services and their careers within the services.

In focusing on the discourses psychology both produces and partakes of, therefore, we are highlighting their motivated, contingent and ideological basis (as opposed to being natural and inevitable). But we are also concerned to identify opportunities for intervening in and changing psychology. While the 'deconstructive' move in psychology is associated with critique rather than the production of alternative constructions, this book moves from a focus in Part I ('Instituting agencies') on identifying the limits and problems with existing practices, to in Part II ('Practicing (at) the limits of representation'), explicitly attending to questions of engagement and conflict within dominant professional discourses at the level of professional practice. Part III ('Dis/ locating institutional boundaries') offers a more sustained consideration of political and conceptual frameworks to recognize and promote resistance.

These frameworks could promote the elaboration of alternative discourses or highlight existing positions of resistance within the institutions of which psychology partakes. In this book we do not provide the conventional (scientific and everyday) narrative of problem posed and then resolved; rather, our aim is to offer some space for the production of new positions and subjectivities. That is, rather than making specific recommendations or prefiguring specific interventions, we challenge the assumptions that have structured the terrain of the 'psy complex', and thus render it open to new possibilities. The postscripts summarize some enduring/emerging conceptual issues and political tensions that have figured in our discussions and now appear in different ways within individual chapters.

Theoretical resources

We draw on four main theoretical resources in this book: deconstruction, Foucauldian analyses, psychoanalysis and discussions of postmodernism. Importing these ideas into psychology from social theory and cultural studies supplements the discussions about language and practice emerging in psychology from 'the crisis'. Thus the 'turn to language' which accompanied the 'new paradigm' as a response to 'the crisis' in psychology has now acquired a deconstructive twist so that the critical and political effects of the crisis themselves become open to deconstruction (see Parker, 1989; Burman, 1996). The term deconstruction refers to a specific methodology associated with the work of Jacques Derrida (e.g. Derrida, 1976; Spivak, 1988) which demonstrates how dominant cultural categories rely on repressed oppositions. Deconstruction works to highlight the cultural and conceptual organization of modern Western thinking around gendered and racialized polarities; and this approach has informed critical discourse work in psychology. Alongside other resources such as social constructionism, this has been used to challenge psychology's claims to offer enduring universal truths (Burman and Parker, 1993). Rather, psychological knowledge is shown to be provisional, partial and ideological. This work explores the relationship between psychological knowledge and the context in which it is produced and deployed. It remains agnostic or even antithetical to the possibility of reforming or improving on psychology.

Second, notwithstanding its eclectic conceptual resources and political ambiguities, a key reference point for this book is the work of Michel Foucault. While Foucault's writings elaborate a range of approaches and preoccupations that variously inform the chapters in this book, we draw on them as a common reference point. His analyses of the emergence of institutions and systems of thinking structuring modern Western societies are especially relevant to the practices in which psychology participates (e.g. Foucault, 1961, 1973, 1977a, 1979b). While Foucauldian analyses cannot be 'applied' in any easy or wholesale way to psychology – such would be antithetical to both the ideas and the conception of psychological practices they give rise to – they are helpful in promoting critical scrutiny of the historical and cultural specificity of the categories and systems that are so integral to modern, Western structures of thinking that they have acquired a felt reality, as 'second nature'. From Foucault's 'histories of the present' we can reflect on how 'reason' and 'madness' are counterposed to each other (as discussed in Chapter 2, and returned to in relation to its gendered inflections in Chapters 5 and 6), how gender and sexuality have come to be constituted as identities rather than positions or activities (the implications of which are discussed in Chapter 10 in relation to the criteria and practices employed by gender identity clinics in regulating sex-change operations), and how particular familial forms and relationships are privileged and others pathologized (taken up in Chapter 8 in relation to discourses of 'mothering').

Developing such analyses, we can begin to explore the consequences of the current arrangement of discourses; how they interrelate and how they conflict, shift and mutate. This attention to the discursive construction of (psychological) practices wards off the relativistic reading of discourses as *merely* social constructions floating free of material practices. We therefore selectively draw upon, but maintain a realist suspicion of, some of the social constructionist work currently gaining popularity in psychology (e.g. Kvale, 1992). While social constructionism enables attention to the multiplicity, it can present each 'story' as equally viable and each position as unconstrained: that is, it denies or underestimates how power relations inform and produce the stories on offer. On the other hand, partly by virtue of this liberal, voluntaristic hue, it does retain some notion of agency – both normative and transgressive – that is theorized and drawn upon at different points in this book in diverse ways. Thus Chapter 2 claims the subject produced by popular self-help books as a site for resistance against the regulatory mental health practices they popularize, while Chapter 10 highlights the forms of subjectivity emerging through and against the new technologies of psychosexual surgery. The tensions between deconstructionism and social constructionism play themselves out in this book between the different projects of commenting on the production and consequences of particular categories (as in the emergence of 'sexual abuse' as an arena of expert knowledge, Chapter 6) and of elaborating new ways of interpreting and engaging with these categories (Chapters 2, 3, 5 and 10). We use Foucault's work to afford a sensitivity to how specific material practices engage with – in the sense of maintaining or disrupting – broader regulatory discourses. We return to the significance of specificity below.

A third key resource for the analyses we present here is psychoanalysis. Psychology has long claimed that a special relationship operates between its agents and objects of study. As embodied (classed, 'raced', gendered, aged, sexed) people researching on or with (depending on your model of psychology) other people, a necessary reflexivity exists. While typically this reflexivity is treated as potential incursions of subjective 'bias' that need to be warded off and erased (as indicated by the work on 'experimenter effects' or 'demand characteristics', cf. Banister *et al.*, 1994), psychoanalytic concepts highlight not only the inevitability of, and neccessity for, such subjective investments, but also permit systematic elaboration of these as a key tool to understand the workings of personal and institutional relationships. Wendy Hollway (1989), in her critique of positivist methodology, deconstructs the traditional opposition between objectivity and subjectivity in psychology (with its corresponding value tags of objective-good/subjective-bad) and argues that objectivity is a particular (and particularly deluded) form of subjectivity. In this book we draw on a psychoanalytically informed understanding of reflexivity, especially in Chapters 3 and 4, as a means of reflecting on research and professional practices, particularly in relation to the strategies used to negotiate and deal with the power relations in which practitioners are inserted. And in Chapter 9 the psychoanalytic ideas of Lacan and Kristeva are combined with the discourse model of Bakhtin to explore the investments in, and transgressive possibilities of, joking relations. But the subscription to psychoanalytic ideas itself comes in for some reflexive scrutiny in Chapter 4, where the project and practice of feminist psychotherapy is subjected to political critique using discourse analysis.

Finally, our focus on the historical construction of psychology locates it within the modern Western project of the Enlightenment, with science, reason and progress as its key triple rhetorical spires (e.g. Flax, 1990). The deconstructive and Foucauldian approach to discourse used in this book takes issue with these tenets of modernity and draws in Chapters 9 and 10 on discussions of postmodernism as a counterpart to the rational unitary individual that underpins modern State institutional practices and which is produced and regulated by psychology. We take up some features of postmodernist accounts to attend to the multiplicity and fluidity of identities and positions (Butler, 1993a; Bhavnani and Haraway, 1994), as a prompt towards envisioning scope for dissonance in and dissidence from psychological discourses.

Regulation and resistance

The dynamic of this book traces a movement from a primary preoccupation with practices of regulation, to attending to the means of elaborating resistance. In Part III, 'Dis/locating institutional boundaries', the postmodern predilection for play and excess combines with a psychoanalytic understanding of contradiction to fuel resistance. But, following Foucault's analyses, regulation and resistance should not be thought of as opposed in any simple way – with regulation as 'bad' and resistance 'good'. While Foucault's account of power is itself not fixed, a sustained theme of this work explores how power is not the unidimensional exercise of authority wielded by one party over another (Foucault, 1980a, 1982; Martin, 1988). Rather, power produces effects which necessarily include resistance. Accordingly, it is sometimes difficult to distinguish between regulation and resistance, as illustrated in Chapter 2 where self-help texts on depression can be read either as liberatory guides dispensing with medical experts, or alternatively as reinforcing discourses of personal responsibility and deference to medical and moral definitions of health and illness – whereby self-help can transmute into self-regulation.

On the other hand, and paradoxically, the very technologies that at broader institutional levels, subordinate and pathologize deviations from the standards that they manufacture (cf. Rose, 1985, 1989) can at more local levels function to promote resistance to them. While educational psychology is often seen (not least by its practitioners) as a prime example of State policing and regulation of working-class children, Chapter 3 discusses how the assertion of professional status within existing hierarchies can be used to empower the most disadvantaged parties in the network of relations: that is, the young people in whose interests the interventions are supposedly, but are rarely actually, made. This chapter also highlights how the practice of testing can also be used to challenge teachers' and parents' perceptions of young people's (in)abilities.

So if regulation can turn into resistance, are practices of resistance of equivalent political ambiguity? If, as in Foucauldian analyses, power produces resistance, then resistance functions in relation to the operations of power and can therefore be complicit in maintaining them (for a clear account of this interplay between constraints and empowerment in relation to knowledge/power, see de Lauretis, 1989). In the discussion of the normalizing practices of gender identity clinics in Chapter 10 we explore the position of transsexuals as a site of resistance to the dominant sex/gendered organization of subjectivity. But, as we conclude there, there are ways in which this can work to reassert rather than resist the existing gendered order. This can occur in two ways: first, through the censorship and self-censorship of accomplished 'passers' through the system so that the fit between the expectations of transsexual identity and experience is secured; and second, because the plurality and variability that new technologies of gender make possible are themselves vulnerable to exploitation by the market which treats them as commodities available for consumption. The ambiguities surrounding the evaluation of resistance come in for systematic treatment in Chapter 8 where responses to dominant discourses of familial forms and mothering are analysed. Here resistance is shown to lie within the act of reading as well as within the texts produced or read. But we would not want to read every reaction as a coherent resistance. And although perspectives vary at different points in the book, we strongly maintain the need for forms of resistance that are collective and organized, rather than individual and spontaneous. In this we depart from some readings of Foucault.

In this sense, the concern with gender issues in Part III reflects the particularly acute relation between feminist and Foucauldian analyses. While Foucault's ideas are attractive because of their clear engagement with discussions of power and institutional practices, feminist analyses have been particularly important in applying and critiquing both his work and poststructuralism generally (cf. Weedon, 1987; Sawicki, 1991; Butler, 1993a; Elam, 1994). While this is not the place to go into specific feminist evaluations of Foucault (see Diamond and Quinby, 1988; Fraser, 1989; McNay, 1992; Ramazanoglu, 1992) or poststructuralism (e.g. Brodribb, 1992), including black and post-colonial critiques (Spivak, 1988), the focus on gender in this final section of the book befits its status as a key arena in which the politics of resistance has been debated.

But, equally, this should not be taken to imply that this is the only part of the book addressing gender issues. Nor that consideration of gender is, as is sometimes conventionally assumed, necessarily about women and still less that gender is monolithic. The children who form the basis of our analysis of school exclusions in Chapter 7 are, significantly, primarily boys, and the gendered and classed patterning of referrals to educational psychologists forms the basis for Chapter 2. In Chapter 5, the absent presence of black women in mental health services is discussed in relation to the racialization of gender, such that 'femininity' has, through colonial and imperial histories, been primarily allocated to white women.

Throughout the book, therefore, the theme of gender arises in terms of gender *relations*. Hence Chapter 5 analyses how the particular configurations of 'race' and gender which produce the overrepresentation of African–Caribbean men gives rise to the corresponding absence of, and exclusions of provision for, African–Caribbean women within the mental health services. Chapter 6 develops this further in terms of the ways stereotypical gender norms enter into the admissions criteria for special hospitals, such that women are considered 'dangerous' on the basis of less serious offences than men. Finally, in Chapter 10, the terms and technologies that maintain 'normal' and 'transgressive' gendered and sexed oppositions (of male/female; and heterosexual/homosexual) themselves are treated as effects of regulatory practices.

Objects and subjects

Having now outlined key features of our framework, we return to their specific exhibition in this book. Discourses and the practices that perform them construct objects. They constitute 'problems' which become the targets of our interventions. Some of these (discussed in this book) are categories of people: black men and women (Chapter 5), sexually abused women (Chapter 6), single mothers (Chapter 8), naughty boys (Chapter 7). Others are entities such as 'depression' (Chapter 2), 'special educational needs' (Chapter 3). What is important here is that both the categories of identities and the entities are wrought by and through the discourses into a very material and subjective reality.

One important contribution of Foucauldian analyses is to highlight that we are as subject to the discourses when they do not appear to speak to, or

Erica Burman

'interpellate', us as when they do. This is because institutions of classification and segregation (such as clinical and educational psychology) regulate those at its centre through its practices of normalization as much as those pathologized targets that fall foul of their boundaries. In this sense, the distinction between object and subject becomes tenuous. However, we take experience, or subjectivity, as both constructed *and* as amenable to direction and application. That is, just because institutions govern and organize our experiences does not mean that we cannot and do not work with, through and against them. Since they are necessarily exposed to the interpretive work we engage in as participants, this is always a site open to variability. In these times of political apathy and resignation amid privatization and the dismantling of the welfare state, finding ways to mobilize (individual and collective) 'agencies' – constructed or not – in the form of resistances is urgent and necessary.

In this book we engage with these double positions of object and subject by drawing on our own varying positions as participants in the practices we discuss. We describe patient, client or service recipient (depending on the practice and model of practice) subjectivities. We analyse the corresponding subject positions elaborated for the practitioners. At times the analysis moves from the general to the specific, with analyses of particular experiences or involvement in case histories. Here experience is taken as a resource to be interrogated – in relation to the role of the educational psychologist in Chapter 3, of the therapist in Chapter 4 and of the researcher in Chapter 7. While a product of historical and immediate practices, experience can nevertheless be used (rather than dismissed as construction or false consciousness) to inform analysis. Moreover, as illustrated in Chapter 2, historical shifts of experience can be mobilized as contrasting positions from which to evaluate contemporary discourses and the analyses of them.

Topics and textualities; structures and specificities

The concept of contradiction has already been mentioned as central to the elaboration of positions of resistance. The subjective textualities explored in this book are reflected in its range of material as well as topics. Chapters are based on interview material (Chapters 6 and 7), 'clinical', 'expert' and 'lay' texts (Chapters 5, 3 and 2 respectively), newspapers and popular cultural sources (Chapters 8 and 9) and on the reflexive analysis of professional practice (Chapters 3, 4, 5 and 7). The role of the material form, or textuality, of the performance of discursive practices itself becomes a topic in Chapter 10.

A focus on textuality contributes to an attention to agencies afforded by discourses. Discourses may position us, but we also perform those positions. Even as we are embedded within structures, the textual features of that enrolement or enactment may permit glimpses of instability or alternative positionings. Thus we need to attend not only to what is written about in magazines or depicted on comic shows, but also how it is read. This kind of analysis reflects the general movement from author to reader in cultural and literary theory (cf. Barthes, 1977). We follow that move here to intimate strategies of resistance and also to highlight how psychological discourses are themselves technologies that produce forms of subjectivity that can resist as well as be regulated.

The attention to specificity as well as structure therefore wards off a monolithic conception of discourses grinding and clashing together to erase agency and accord subjectivity the status of mere effect. While subjectivity is an effect or construction of prevailing classed and racialized discourses of personal responsibility, rational citizenship, gender and sexuality (to take some of the examples we discuss here), this does not mean that it is *only* an effect. Constructed in origin or not, these effects (and affects) are currently all too real. That is, in various chapters subjectivity is taken as a resource to be problematized, while in others it is treated as mobilizing a set of agencies that, albeit constructed, can act. Similarly, within a discursive understanding of its particular and social construction, some chapters draw on specific experiences with a singular narrative voice, while others speak more generally. But we use individual experience not (or not only) as confession, but as a practical means for analysing and countering the workings of institutions.

On the other hand, attending to the multiple political valences of the specific and the general, or the personal and the practice, invites a wariness against setting up another opposition in which global structure equals bad and local textuality equals good. As we have already indicated, the complexity of local–global discursive relations resists such simple allocations, as also that between construction and agent. The specific case can be just as much an instance of regulation as the distal structures that called it forth.

Interventions

This book applies discourse perspectives to psychological practices. In doing so it makes interventions within those practices. This arises from the interdisciplinarity of bringing a range of critical frameworks from outside psychology to bear on our work. It also facilitates a corresponding *intra*-disciplinarity, coordinating the frequently divided arenas of theory, method and practice. Moreover, this also brings about other specific interventions.

In terms of methodological developments, we highlight the usefulness of Foucault's genealogical approach and the discussions this has generated. In particular, we can use these to analyse how the practices we participate in, and that form the fabric of our personal and professional lives, have come to adopt their current shape(s). We demonstrate the importance of interrogating not only how certain constructs have come to be privileged, but also the interpretive and political value of interrogating the absences or silences in this conceptual landscape. Finally, we offer analytical strategies and practical examples to inform engagement with the power relations that imbricate our activity, and highlight agencies to negotiate with these.

For this project we offer some conceptual interventions within existing discourse approaches. Many of the chapters adopt the strategy of formulating counter-discourses in opposition to prevailing institutional practices. These emerge from an attention to the gaps in discourses, whether arising from interpreting the silences in policy or from reading between and beyond the lines of interview transcripts, self-help texts, and even to explore investments and reactions mobilized in professional relations. In Chapter 10, we develop the concept of 'boundary object' as formulated from ethnographic work in institutional and organizational settings exploring communication and coordinating technologies (Star and Griesemer, 1989; Star, 1991). We use this to treat psychological theories, practices and technologies as varieties of conceptual objects which mediate, as well as mark, the boundaries between contested and regulated subjectivities.

Finally, this book can also function as a boundary object: as a text, it is itself a part of the technologies it comments on, but it may afford new relations and possibilities. Our engagement in writing this book is premised on a shared commitment to do more than reinscribe the positions we hold. In writing this, we analyse and develop discussions about these positions, to afford the emergence of additional perspectives. As a co-authored text, this book is itself the outcome of multiple discourses and subjectivities. No rational unitary subject lies behind this text and we are in alliance with Curt (1994) in challenging the official norms of univocality and individual scholarship presumed in academic research. While in this chapter we adopt a common subject position, marked by the pronoun 'we', elsewhere we shift between singular and plural (but organized) authorship. In this chapter we want to highlight this combination of collective and singular voices as a performative example of the socially mediated and multiple textualities that have enabled its production. Each chapter in this book is the outcome of individual research, prompted by personal and professional commitment, investment, positioning. Both as individuals and as a group, we are not uniform subjectivities and the precise arrangement of theoretical influences and political engagements displayed here has emerged through our discussions, agreements and disagreements. Some of the tensions and debates generated through this process are elaborated in the postscripts. Here we want to make clear that, as with our topics, we as authors, as subjects, cannot erase the conflict, nor can we claim or wish to claim a spurious harmony or unity for this book. Nevertheless, we present this account as offering a range of fruitful ways of understanding the oppressive practices we seek to disrupt, unsettle and change, and of forming new alliances and collectivities, even as it has for us.

Part I

Instituting agencies

The three chapters in this section are linked together by the authors' attention to deconstructing the polarized dualisms of the notions of regulation and resistance within and about psychology as discourse and social practice. It emerges that it is neither possible nor desirable to separate author and subject, mind and body, self and institution or professional and lay expert, as oppositional characters, victims and hero(ines) within this postmodern narrative. However, each chapter has a main protagonist whose tale acts to symbolize and highlight particular story lines whose function is to document the myriad of subject positions which are available to critics of psychology and critical psychologists who wish to intervene in its practice and discourse. In this section, the focus is on children, women and emotions, all of which have been and continue to be seen by psychology as needing control. In constructing their stories, the authors seek to make available further positions for disrupting the 'psychological complex' (Rose, 1985).

Allwood's analysis of self-help literature on depression in Chapter 2 looks at the issue of intervention from what might be thought of as an oppositional stance to that of the professional expert. This chapter demonstrates how 'becoming an expert on oneself' draws on the very concepts which inform and uphold those professional bastions such as psychiatry or psychology, which it seeks to circumvent. This literature also invites the adoption of prevalent liberal, humanistic discourses of the agentic and responsible subject 'self'. In contrast to 'self as expert', Billington in Chapter 3 offers a history of the development of the profession of educational psychologists which both depended on as well as elaborated the characteristics of the category 'children', deeming them uncontrollable and in need of 'caring' intervention from the State. By virtue of the insertion of psychological discourse into the institution of education, the status of the psychologist as expert carer and regulator is made possible. However, the function of this expert may not be absolutely fixed, in that it is possible to utilize the tools of the trade for the benefit of the child. This involves both appropriating these tools in order to challenge adopted practices and opening up the practices available to the educational psychologist to include, in this instance, psychodynamic therapeutic tools. Themes from the first two chapters are taken up in Chapter 4 by Heenan, on the subject of feminist therapy. Like educational psychology and the self-help literature, feminist therapy constructs its own discourses (about women and 'women's problems') but without recognizing that it draws unquestioningly on discourses of feminism and psychotherapy, thereby reproducing that which it wants to change. By discursively analysing a feminist clinical supervision of an eating problems psychotherapy group, Heenan explicates ways in which the therapists draw on particular notions of feminism, women and therapy which inform therapeutic practice.

Far from reading this section as a pessimistic account of the pervasiveness of discourse, there is a twist to each chapter's tale whereby disentangling the discursive nature of resistive as well as regulatory practices offers the possibility of a more optimistic reading, even one which lends itself to possibilities for action.

Chapter 2

'I have depression, don't I?':
Discourses of help and self-help books

Robin Allwood

Caveat emptor (Let the buyer beware)

Between writing the penultimate and final drafts of this chapter I experienced another bout of depression. In terms of rhetorical strategy I have several reasons for mentioning this. First, I want to suggest that what follows is part of a continuing personal struggle to develop a partial understanding of experiences that have had a profound impact on my life. Second, I might want to claim some form of 'expert' status and deflect attention from my investment in this work as part of a future doctoral thesis.

Finally and, with regard to the content of this chapter, most substantively, I want to highlight the ease with which, by my writing and your reading, we are able to collude in the creation of an objectified thing called 'depression'; to reify a descriptively elusive way of experiencing situated in the particular circumstances of someone's life. It's almost as though the experience could be held up to one's gaze and, thus interrogated, be made to give up its generic secrets and universal properties. Thus we must ask how our metaphors for a way of being, for example, Churchill's 'black dog' or a list of 'symptoms', simultaneously assist and occlude our understanding.

Introduction

> Books on depression are rarely enlightening.
> Dorothy Rowe, *The Experience of Depression*

The experience of 'depression' causes great distress both to the individual and to their friends and family. Rowe (1983) argues that the key point in coping with this distress is to 'understand what is happening to you' (p. 263). This understanding is often sought by consulting 'self-help' books available from bookshops and local libraries. But the advice and instruction about how to deal with 'depression' offered in this form of popular psychology is neither consistent nor unproblematic. In this chapter I adopt a social constructionist approach to this multiplicity of ways of accounting. The critical problem I address is the complex relationship between notions of personal empower-ment and self-regulation. Through an analysis of the discourses of self-help, I examine a variety of concepts of 'depression', deconstructing them in an attempt to uncover some of the hidden issues around the ideas of help (medi-cal) and self-help (personal). With regard to the question of self-regulation I suggest a discourse analysis can help inform strategies of personal and societal resistance by problematizing the dominant medical construction of 'depres-sion' and so regenerating space for the expression and appreciation of alterna-tive points of view.

The conceptualization of 'depression'

Foucault's (1961) investigation of the social construction of madness highlights the mutability and variety of cultural understandings of 'mental illness'. But how does one generate a concept of, for example, 'depression'? The first step is to translate experiences grounded in the unique and particular circum-stances of someone's life by giving those experiences a name. Butler (1993b) calls this practice *performativity*: 'that aspect of discourse that has the capacity to produce what it names' (p. 33). Alternatively, in Fromm's (1979) terms, this 'sleight of mind' reifies a way of *being* into a way of *having*: I *am* depressed becomes I *have* depression.

The second step is to define the concept, which raises the question of who is accorded the knowledge/power to perform such a delimitation. Within psychiatric literature the classification of 'depression' is a continuing source of debate and confusion (Farmer and McGuffin, 1989) although the *right* of the psychiatric profession to define depression is not called into question. In this chapter I argue that 'depression' is a concept that is polymorphously socially constructed. By this I mean that each account of 'depression' that an author formulates in their text is contingent on their situated and motivated aims and objectives.

Given this multiplicity of descriptions of 'depression', it is possible, first, to look for areas where its definition is contested and, second, to analyse an author's particular construction in terms of the discourses employed and the power relations both within and between them. The popular literary genre of self-help books constitutes a key arena where a variety of definitions of 'de-pression' are offered to the general public and questions of experience, agency and responsibility, are elaborated and contested.

Self-help and self-regulation

Self-help books on 'depression' offer accessible accounts of mainstream (malestream) psychological theories and practices. Theorists following the Foucauldian tradition adopt a critical stance towards mainstream psychology, for example Rose (1985, 1989). These, in addition to feminist theorists keen to address a self-help genre which has been seen as mainly directed towards women (as in diet programmes) provide two interesting viewpoints with which to discuss the notions of self-help and self-regulation. However, it should be noted that, just as regulation and resistance should not be simplistically treated as oppositional qualities, we must not imagine self-help and self-regulation as the poles of another theoretical dualism. Rather, the designation of a discourse, or one of its elements, as regulatory or helpful, or both, is made possible by virtue of a motivated discursive entity performing that judgement within a specific social context.

Nikolas Rose's (1989) work elaborates the Foucauldian notion of self-regulation. Rose argues that experts, as mediators between the State and the individual, use their expertise to educate the individual into a self-critical and self-regulatory mode of being. This is done through a conjunction of the establishment of 'facts', the inducement of personal anxiety about deviation from social 'norms' and the promise of a happier self with a better future in prospect. The latter quality is of particular relevance to those of us who experience being depressed; each of the texts to be examined below contains an attractive vision of what life *could* be like, usually when one has thoroughly enacted the techniques and practices advocated. As Rose (1989) says: '[b]ehaviour modification . . . is easily transformed into a technique of self-analysis and self-help . . . into a pathway to asserting ourselves' (p. 237). In terms of national government, or the 'State', self-regulation assists the unsystematic 'reorganization' of medical services: why seek help from a State, publicly-funded psychologist (or private practitioner) when you can do-it-yourself?

Schilling and Fuehrer (1993), working from a critical feminist standpoint, argue that the 'self-help' book genre 'is aimed primarily at women' (p. 418) in that it deals with 'difficulties most epidemiological analyses would classify as "women's problems" (depression, weight and anxiety problems)' (p. 418). Further, whereas Cheal (1991) specifies 'lack of confidence in experts' (p. 150) as a major characteristic of postmodern society, Schilling and Fuehrer note that 'rather than disrupting relationships of power through broad dissemination of knowledge, this popularization [of psychology] appears to have strengthened the rhetorical stance of the expert' (p. 418). Thus an issue of importance for the analysis below is the practices authors use to position relations between themselves and the reader.

Two further issues raised by feminist criticism revolve around the possibility of the damaging effects arising from the liberal humanist model that often underlies therapeutic theory. First, Coward (1989) points out that '[w]e live in a society which believes the individual is responsible for his or her actions and indeed that the individual is ultimately responsible for whatever happens to her in society, whether she succeeds or fails' (p. 199). Thus, if we repeatedly experience being depressed, we will not only be unhappy, but we can blame ourselves, our weak personality, our lack of willpower, etc. What is intended as an empowering philosophy can potentially make one more of a victim. So I must ask: for the person who experiences being depressed, what are the consequences of the various understandings offered in terms of causes identified, treatments suggested and the possibility of a cure?

The second point concerns the implications for social and societal change. It has been noted that liberal humanism posits the notion of a 'natural' or 'true' self within each of us and so 'leads directly and inevitably to the idea of *personal* solutions and *individual* liberation' (Scott and Payne, 1984: p. 22; my emphasis). Schilling and Fuehrer (1993), while welcoming the recognition of the 'oppressive condition of women's lives', also do not want to see the need for a 'restructuring of social arrangements' subsumed in an exclusive focus on 'personal development' (p. 418). While broadly agreeing with this view, I would argue that a person who is depressed may well have to focus on individual solutions before addressing a wider perspective. Finally, it is worth pointing out that I affirm the agency of the reader, for example the pragmatic or strategic ability to appropriate useful practices from a text without adopting its ideological content. But here I am concerned with offering my own deconstructive reading of self-help texts, via a discourse analysis, so my focus is on exposing the persuasive strategies adopted by the authors themselves.

Discourse analysis

While discourse, in the sense of the institutional structuring of subjectivity, forms a key theme of this book, I will confine myself here to a brief discussion of the practical issues that will be raised in the following analysis. First, as Burman and Parker (1993) state, discourse analysis has brought the work of the French philosopher, Michel Foucault, into social psychology 'to provide a critical account of the function of the discipline of psychology itself' (p. 7). An example of this is Rose's notion of self-regulation mentioned above. Second, a discourse analytic approach to psychology 'works to highlight the assumptions underlying [psychological accounts] and challenges their facticity, that is, their status as truth' (Burman and Parker, 1993, p. 8). Thus, a feature of my analysis will be to highlight the ways in which the 'fact' that 'depression is a mental illness' is proposed and contested. Third, there is a concern with the issue of reflexivity at all points in the research process. This 'self-conscious attention' on the part of discourse analysts promotes consideration of questions of accountability and interpretation in the presentation of research findings. Further, it works to make evident the implicit power relations structured in texts, for example between the researcher and the researched, the writer and the reader. This standpoint has two practical implications in what follows: i) an account of the theoretical structure of discourse adopted, and ii) an attention to the different ways authors, including myself, construct their 'expert' status within the text.

Although it by no means necessarily does this, discourse analysis can 'be taken up in useful ways to inform political struggles' (Burman and Parker, 1993, p. 10) by proponents of varying political persuasions. Thus, any definition or structure used to represent discourse is contingent on the author's, or speaker's, purposes as well as the available cultural resources. In developing the version of discourse used here, I draw on Parker (1992) who points out that the acknowledgment of reflexivity in discourse analysis enables a grounded attention to the qualities of ideology, social structures (institutions) and social relations (practices and power relations). In this analysis of 'self-help' texts I focus in particular on an examination of ideology. This is because it is the author's encoded ideology which attempts to interpellate the reader as the 'self', i.e. as the institution of personal discourse, and to urge them to adopt certain strategies or practices.

On a final reflexive note, I draw the reader's attention to my use of conceptual devices and rhetorical strategies in constructing the analysis. I, no less than the authors whose work I discuss, render a partial and motivated account; an account which is but one of a multiplicity of possible readings and thus by no means definitive or veridical in any absolute sense.

Introducing the texts

The five books selected for the analysis were drawn from a town-centre library catalogue where they were classified under the heading 'depression'. These were as follows (see Appendix on page 36 for references): first, Goldberg (1984) who defines depression as a 'psychological illness' and presents an orthodox medical account of help and self-help in a 'question and answer' format; second, Lake (1987) who argues that the origin of depression lies in damaging socialization techniques adopted by those in parental roles and thus he offers a series of new strategies to be enacted in social interactions with people who still attempt to manipulate the individual in these ways; third, McRae (1986) who gives an autobiographical account of her experience of depression in the late 1960s, during which she underwent a period of psychoanalysis; fourth, Priest (1983) regards depression as an abnormal medical condition and gives a 'step by step' guide to issues such as self-diagnosis, when to seek medical advice, the effects of prescribed drugs, etc.; and, finally, Rowe (1983) who contends that depression is the result of a personal moral judgement on the self related to a decision to maintain a set of erroneous opinions about oneself and others.

The practice of discourse analysis involves close textual examination. It was therefore necessary to select a topic or issue whose presentation and treatment could be analysed in the various texts. I was particularly interested to see how authors constructed their definitions and descriptions of 'depression': three of the texts had chapters headed 'What is depression?', McRae's fourth chapter was entitled 'Depression', and I was able to look at the fifth, Rowe's, version using the first chapter ('The Prison') and the first section of

Chapter 3 ('How to build your prison'). In addition to these five texts, I included a newer book by Pitt (1993) in the analysis because it was produced as part of the 'Defeat Depression' campaign, organized jointly by the Royal Colleges of Psychiatrists and General Practitioners (RCP and RCGP), with the avowed aim of increasing public awareness about 'depression'. It is interesting to note that the British Psychological Society (BPS) seems not to have been invited to participate formally in the campaign but then, whatever else it may be, depression is represented as exclusively a *medical* problem (see discussion of medical ideology below).

The analysis

My analysis below is split into two parts: a discussion of i) an educational meta-discourse that overarches the entire 'self-help' genre, and ii) the four discourses identified within the texts that most closely touch on the themes of regulation and resistance.

An educational meta-discourse

The supposed democracy of the child-centred pedagogy (Walkerdine and Lucey, 1989), with its corresponding production of self-regulating citizens, is here enacted by the market through the exercise of 'choice' over the consumption of goods. The school, the usual socially designated institution of educational discourse, is replaced by a collaboration between author and book publisher who now provide the educational material. Thus a self-help text is the constructed pedagogical product of an individual and an institution; both of which have a business interest in the commercial performance of the text as a product of the self-help industry. This implicit agenda is mentioned in only one text, Pitt (1993), and then in an oblique fashion: 'But mainly this book has been written for . . . the masses (if we are lucky)' (p. viii). Elsewhere in this book (Chapter 9) we touch on the multiple themes of regulation and resistance expressed by jokes. Here I simply want to note that the self-help genre relies on the liberal model of society as organized around free and separate agents interacting through market relations.

In terms of the ideology of education, three types of target audience were typically identified by the writers, e.g. Lake (1987, p. 7):

> This book has been written for three groups of people. The first consists of those who suffer directly from depression, and are puzzled and perplexed by it and want to know what to do to feel better. The second, are people who are concerned about somebody else who is depressed and would like to know more about how to help. And

third are those who want to be better informed generally about the subject.

Depending on whether the reader identifies themselves as a sufferer, helper or general interest reader, the reader is interpellated within the educational discourse as someone who is 'puzzled', 'wants to know more' or 'be better informed'. The writer is correspondingly positioned as an expert who can provide this information. However, different writers focused on different target groups, e.g. Pitt (1993) says 'mainly this book has been written for the general public' (p. viii). On the other hand, Lake (1987, p. 7) states:

> Although the book is about depression and sets out to explain why people become depressed, its main purpose is not to describe the problem, but to explain in practical terms what to do to solve it.

Thus Lake's focus is on the 'sufferer' and his expertise will provide a practice, i.e. a method to be enacted. 'Depression' is conceived within educational ideology as a 'practical problem' that can be 'explained' and so 'solved'.

The social relations of educational discourse offer two positions: teacher and student. The question posed by several authors as a chapter heading, i.e. 'What is depression?', indicates the writer's construction of themselves as the teacher who knows *the* answer (note the singular) and will explain it to the reader/student (by contrast I have already indicated that I am a student and, at the risk of destroying the narrative of suspense, I can reveal here that I have no great revelations about the experience of being depressed to offer you). The motivation of the reader/student who is also a 'sufferer' is to gain an understanding of depression and learn a methodology that will prevent its recurrence. Lake (1987) is quite outspoken in his view that 'depression is something we have to defeat completely. No other objective is acceptable' (p. 7). Note that the teacher and student are located on the same side in Lake's battle metaphor. This formulation ignores the unequal power relations of the teacher/student dyad (shades here of the suppression of power conflicts within 'democratic' discourse). Also, should the reader 'lose' the 'battle', they are consequently positioned as a poor student and a weak fighter: 'must try harder'.

This didactic relationship is expressed in the writer/teacher's practice of presenting their argument in the 'question and answer' format already noted in the use of chapter headings. Rowe (1983) also presents the reader with questions such as 'What is the difference between being depressed and unhappy?' (p. 1) and 'How can you describe this experience and convey its meaning to someone else?' (p. 2). Squire's (1990, p. 39) discussion of the use of the detective narrative in social psychology texts is relevant here:

> by setting up a problem, an unresolved crime, and resolving it, step by step, it crystallises narrative's interest in logical completeness, or closure.

Thus Goldberg (1984), as writer/teacher and now detective, solves the 'mystery' of depression with the closure '[it is] a psychological illness' (p. 6). Goldberg's fifth reason for calling depression an 'illness' is that:

> despite the carping criticisms of some less thoughtful medical sociologists, it is much less *stigmatising* to be thought depressed than to be thought guilty of some moral crime. The medical standpoint is morally neutral. (p. 6)

The criticisms of 'some medical sociologists' are those of people who are fault-finding, peevish and fond of taking exception. Goldberg trivializes and dismisses the argument of agents within medical discourse who don't share his point of view. Squire (1990) also points out that the detective is an enemy 'of any moral order' which produces criminals (or crimes). Thus, as Goldberg sees it, some medical sociologists are thoughtlessly supporting the view of depression as a moral crime. Whereas he, by asserting the 'moral neutrality' of medical discourse, is benignly decriminalizing depression, removing stigma by labelling depression an 'illness', i.e. an object of medical discourse. In this way Goldberg constructs and defends his 'facts' about depression.

The power relations set up in self-help texts denote a variety of paired subject positions, for example, writer/reader, teacher/student and detective/victim, which are seldom made explicit. As Squire (1990, p. 40) says:

> social psychological narratives usually differ from detective stories in writing the investigator out . . . But the authority of the absent investigator lies behind every passive textual construction . . . s/he becomes like the detective, the moral reformer guiding the narrative.

At first sight it may seem that McRae's (1986) autobiographical account of her experience of being depressed does not fit into the model of educational discourse. However, her moving account of distress, treatment and recovery may be read as a template for action, guiding the reader/student towards psychotherapy in general and psychoanalysis in particular. McRae's authority does stem from a different source to the other authors. Fromm (1979) distinguishes between '*having* authority and *being* an authority' (p. 44). In Fromm's sense the other authors *have* authority because of their psychological expertise, while McRae *is* an authority by dint of her personal experiences.

Having embedded the following discussion within an educational meta-discourse, I move on to the second part of the analysis: an examination of the four discourses I identified as being most closely related to the themes of regulation and resistance. These discourses – personal, medical, commercial and governmental – will be engaged with under the headings 'social structures', 'competing ideologies' and 'social practices'.

Social structures

Perhaps not surprisingly, all the authors seemed to see the 'self' as the sole site for the elaboration of personal discourse. This self, or unitary rational subject (see Henriques *et al.* (1984) for a critique of this notion), interacts with other institutions such as the family, networks of friends and colleagues in the workplace. For example, McRae (1986, p. 43) describes the personal struggle between her emotional distress and her responsibilities and duties as a health visitor:

> On the day that I returned to work I felt excited, and confident that I would be able to forget the torment of the past few months. I spent the morning reading through the records to see which families needed an urgent visit, and in the afternoon I made a few calls, but at the end of the day my fears and anxieties still remained; they dominated my mind. My confidence was gone.

This focus on the self and personal responsibility is precisely that which, as Schilling and Fuehrer (1993) noted, obscures the need for wider social change.

The most commonly referred to institution of medical discourse in the six texts was the 'general or family practice' with its agent as the general practitioner (GP). At a societal level, McRae's (1986) account touches on the National Health Service (NHS) and private practice, while Pitt (1993) mentions two professional bodies: the RCP and the RCGP. In relation to the 'diagnosis' of depression Pitt also notes an 'American "bible"' (p. 14), used also by many psychiatrists outside the USA, which is how he refers to the *Diagnostic and Statistical Manual of Mental Disorders* (1987, third edition, revised; DSM-III-R) published by the American Psychiatric Association.

A factor affecting the treatment someone who experiences being depressed will receive is the availability of services. At this point, medical discourse intersects with a third discourse: commercial (note that most of the texts used in this analysis were produced prior to the 'break-up' of the NHS into purchasers and providers of services, and fund-holding versus non-fund-holding practices which has since made the commercial discourse much more explicit. It may be that commercial discourse will be more overtly stated in future texts). McRae's (1986) account highlights the difference between two types of medical institution in terms of commercial discourse: i) publicly funded bodies, such as the general practice and the NHS and ii) privately funded bodies, such as Dr Goldblatt's practice as a psychoanalyst.

Finally, in terms of governmental discourse, the institution explicitly concerned with depression at a societal level is the Department of Health (DOH). The DOH exerts influence on medical institutions, such as the RCP and RCGP, through its collation and publication of statistics on the prevalence of depression. These figures define the parameters of the problem nationally by providing baseline 'facts' which are then utilized to produce official improvement 'targets', e.g. *The Health of the Nation* (1993a).

A number of diverse institutions, such as the self, general practice, the Department of Health have been introduced in connection with the management of 'depression' at different levels of society. I now move on to look at how these institutions are orientated towards each other.

Competing ideologies

Overall, two important notions were developed in terms of a personal discourse of the 'self': the 'mind', subdivided into 'emotion' and 'reason', and the 'body'. Taking the mind first, the above extract from McRae illustrates the idea of emotion. The self is the unitary subject which contains and reflects on 'feelings' that are differentiated into categories such as excitement, confidence, torment, fear and anxiety. Later McRae discusses her situation with a friend called Rita:

> 'What are you going to do about it?'
> 'What more can I do?' I asked. 'I'm taking Librium regularly, and I keep telling myself there's no reason why I should be like this, but it doesn't make any difference.' (p. 46)

Rita's question appeals to McRae's sense of personal responsibility and thus invokes a second quality of mind: reason. But McRae replies that her attempts to rationalize her 'state' have been unsuccessful. For McRae the emotional distress she is experiencing is more powerful than her ability to reason with it: 'I was imprisoned in my mind' (p. 49). In this penal metaphor (which generates a judicial discourse also found in Rowe, 1983) McRae is represented as confined in a mind where emotional distress holds sway over the ability to reason.

The notion of reason within personal ideology is treated differently in Rowe (1983, p. 13):

> there are some things in life . . . about which each of us must have an opinion. It is this set of opinions about these aspects of life which determines whether or not we become depressed.

Rowe's emphasis here is on the self's responsibility for the choice to maintain certain opinions which lead to depression. Through the causal chain of:

reason → responsibility → choice → opinions → depression

Rowe argues that the self is exclusively responsible for being depressed and thus the self has power over depression. This argument is an example of the potentially damaging effects of the radical liberal humanism discussed by Coward (1989): a consequence of continuing to experience being depressed can be an impression of personal failure.

A second major quality of personal ideology is the 'body':

> Of course there are physical changes when we are depressed. Every emotion, pleasant or unpleasant, is accompanied by physical changes which become more profound the longer the emotion persists. (p. 13)

This quotation from Rowe (1983) suggests that the mind, through its emotional properties, produces physical changes in the body. This view is vividly described by McRae:

> As I sat alone eating my lunch I felt as though my heart kept missing a beat. I had a sense of foreboding: a sinking feeling inside me. The sensation overwhelmed me like a giant wave on a stormy sea. I jumped up desperate to escape. I rushed around the clinic, trying to relieve the tension, but my panic increased. (p. 44)

Here, ideas of emotion – 'a sense of foreboding' and 'panic' – are related to dualistic notions of the body as that which experiences physical 'sensations' such as a 'sinking feeling' and 'tension'.

Within personal discourse, depression has been diversely constituted in terms of a reasoning and emoting mind and a physical body. Typically, there has been a liberal humanist emphasis on reason and responsibility in promoting *personal* wellbeing which, as I have argued, can have damaging consequences for the individual and which leaves untheorized the role of society.

Considering medical discourse, a frequently used starting-point was to distinguish between what Goldberg (1984, p. 1) describes as 'feelings of sadness' and the 'illness' called depression:

> When doctors speak of depression they mean much more than the experience of sadness. Depression is an abnormal state in which the feelings of sadness are accompanied by numerous other related symptoms which impair efficiency and which do not go away by themselves.

There are a number of points worth noting about this definition: i) the absence of a self that experiences the depression, i.e. it is a 'condition' or 'state'; ii) it is an 'abnormal state' which 'does not correct itself' and so, on both counts, requires a doctor's attention; and iii) it is more than simply 'feelings of sadness' as it is accompanied by 'related symptoms' which 'impair efficiency'. Thus Goldberg uses a medical metaphor of the self that constitutes the body as a biological organism whose abnormal functioning can be recognized by the presence of certain symptoms. For Goldberg the issue of normality/

abnormality is related to the functioning of 'homeostatic mechanisms': that is, self-regulating systems which maintain the body within normal functional parameters. Further, Goldberg extends the idea of self-regulating systems to the consideration of sadness and depression, i.e. sadness can be homeostatically regulated (normal) but in depression this regulatory process has failed (abnormal). Goldberg's construction of depression supplants the personal ideology of the self's emotional distress with a mechanical medical model of an abnormally functioning biological organism.

Later, Goldberg offers a tentative definition of 'health' as a matter of: 'each function of our bodies being inside a normal range with ways of returning function to that range if it is disturbed' (p. 4). So the abnormally functioning biological organism acquires the additional quality of being 'unhealthy'.

Finally, after listing a series of symptoms involving categories such as weight, sleep, energy, motor activity, sexual functions, concentration, thought processes and mood, Goldberg gives a list of 'good reasons for calling a state like this an *illness*' (p. 5) which include: i) normal homeostasis has failed; ii) mortality; iii) morbidity; and iv) positive response to treatment. So, through Goldberg's argument, the experience of being depressed has been reified into a condition which is abnormal, unhealthy and an illness. He concludes: 'Doctors therefore describe her [an hypothetical bereaved mother] as having a psychological illness, and they call the illness depression' (p. 6). This constitutes depression within medical discourse as a psychological illness whose treatment is the province of doctors, as the agents to dispense medical discourse.

Other accounts of medical ideology contrast strongly with Goldberg's elaborate construction of depression as a psychological illness. Pitt (1993) simply states: '[depression] is the most common, overlooked and treatable mental illness' (p. vii). Here there is no question of offering an explanation or justification of depression's status as a 'mental illness': it is a *fact*.

On the other hand, Priest (1983), like Goldberg, distinguishes between the feelings of sadness which generally follow an unpleasant 'life-event' and what he calls 'severe disabling depression'. Priest proposes a scale of depression, in terms of severity and duration, in relation to the magnitude of the 'triggering' life-event. This raises the issue of the means by which one can identify oneself, or another, as being depressed:

> In the end deciding when depression – whether it is ours or somebody else's – is abnormal is a very difficult decision in many cases . . . the best guideline is that when depression begins to take over your life and affect everything adversely, then you may well need help. (p. 19)

In Priest's definition of inefficient functioning, the ability to maintain a coherent discourse of the self marks the point at which the individual should submit to medical discourse. He goes on to list psychological and physical 'symptoms' associated with depression. To aid the reader's self-diagnosis, he points out that both types of symptoms will be experienced heterogeneously in terms of number and severity. So, while constituting depression as an object of medical discourse, Priest highlights the variability of its manifestation. He also introduces the problematic distinction between 'reactive' (exogenous) and 'endogenous' depression. Farmer and McGuffin (1989) note the gradual abandonment of this distinction in the clinical literature; an example of mutability of medical discourse as opposed to its monolithic appearance.

Notwithstanding their differences, therefore, the three constructions of depression discussed above, i.e. Goldberg (1984), Pitt (1993) and Priest (1983), concur in portraying depression as a medical illness that requires treatment by a doctor who in turn may recommend 'specialist help'. Lake (1987) takes this a step further to interpret the practices of medicine as 'services' to be made use of by the individual. While presenting depression as in some sense a 'serious medical illness', Lake argues that:

> What we have to do if we wish to *cure* depression is to look beyond the present orthodox medical treatment of the illness and begin to tackle it for ourselves. (p. 15; my emphasis)

The medical services available are characterized as 'orthodox': that is to say in a pejorative way as mundane or ordinary and as designed to alleviate 'symptoms' rather than achieve a cure. For Lake, a cure for depression is related to a personal understanding of its cause which he argues lies in a system of manipulative techniques used in the socialization of children by those in parental roles. Speaking personally, I do not believe the concept of 'cure' is applicable to the experience of being depressed but, as Lake has introduced it, it is worth noting the difference between his notion of what constitutes a cure, i.e. the enaction of assertive techniques in social situations, and its use in dominant medical discourse where it is understood as the absence of symptoms.

Rowe's (1983) opposition to 'orthodox' medical ideology takes a different form:

> Depression is not a genetic fault or a mysterious illness which descends on us. It is something we create for ourselves, and just as we create it, so we can dismantle it our creation. (sic, p. 13)

Rowe rejects outright the idea that depression is an illness caused by an outside agent, such as a germ, or that it has a genetic component (cf. Gilbert's (1992) biopsychosocial model) and asserts her construction of depression as a personal creation for which the self remains personally responsible.

To summarize so far, from this small sample of 'self-help' texts I have demonstrated the variability of some constructions of depression within medical ideology. This mutability contrasts strongly with, for example, Pitt's (1993) monolithic assertion that depression is a 'treatable mental illness' (p. viii). Statements like this conceal the socially constructed, debated and contested, nature of such matters as systems of classification, analogies between mental and physical states, proposed treatments, etc., in medical discourse.

Turning now to the ideology of commercial discourse, McRae (1986) relates a conversation between her friend, Rita, and McRae's GP:

> Then Rita spoke. 'Don't you think psychotherapy would help her?'
> 'Yes, I do,' he replied. 'She needs psychotherapy, but there's no way of getting it through the National Health Service. I used to be able to refer people to the Tavistock Centre, but they are no longer accepting people from as far afield as this because they've been inundated. In this area there's a two-year waiting list for psychotherapy, so we've no option but to continue with the drugs.'
> 'What about her having psychotherapy privately?'
> 'If she's prepared to spend a lot of money, and if she can find a psychotherapist, then all right, but I don't know of anyone I can recommend.' (p. 47)

Through her medical agent McRae's need for help is constructed in terms of the bureaucratic practicalities of a large publicly-funded institution offering services which are oversubscribed. McRae as a 'patient' is linked to a geographical catchment 'area' which has an allocation of psychotherapeutic services organized through a 'waiting list'. Further, it seems that the medical agent, because of his knowledge of these practicalities, is ethically justified in concealing his opinion that 'she needs psychotherapy'; something it might be better for her to know. This is an example of the practice of 'resource-led definition' where not only treatment, but also diagnosis, is contingent on the availability of resources.

However, as her GP points out, private psychotherapy presents difficulties of availability and funding. Later in the narrative, McRae's friend, Rita, contacts Dr Goldblatt, a specialist medical agent offering psychoanalytic services on a privately funded basis:

> 'Dr Goldblatt is busy, and he has no free time, but he's agreed to see you in his lunch hour on Wednesday . . . You must realise that he hasn't promised he'll treat you, but at least he'll give you an opinion.' (p. 48)

Here McRae's 'case' is passed from her GP (overtly medical discourse but implicitly business discourse as his services are funded through taxation) to a private psychoanalyst (overtly medical and business discourse) via Rita (friendship discourse). Also, Rita has made the point that Dr Goldblatt has stressed that the meeting does not constitute a contract to treat McRae; he has reserved the option to offer/withhold further service.

At the societal level at which the state apparatus functions, the issue of 'depression' is constructed according to statistics of prevalence and practices of prevention. The problem of suicide is translated into a 'target' figure incorporating a time-limit for the reduction nationally of this fatal personal practice. In describing suicide as 'the worst possible outcome of depression', Pitt (1993, p. 12) states that:

> one in seven sufferers from severe depression will eventually die from suicide. In the Department of Health's paper, *The Health of the Nation* (published in 1993a), the aim is to reduce the number of suicides by 15% by the beginning of the next century, which demands a very determined effort to find and treat depressive illness more effectively.

The 'Defeat Depression' campaign can here be seen as an instance of that 'very determined effort to find and treat depressive illness'. Thus government discourse endorses the dominant construction of depression within medical discourse as a 'mental illness'. This reinforcement may become a cause for concern when considering the issue of self-regulation because such a conjunction of powerful social structures can restrict the development of alternative constructions of 'depression', e.g. by controlling the allocation of research funding. Also, by endorsing the medical model, which itself reduces personal distress to (or at best recasts it as) illness, the State can ignore the need for wider social change. This, doubtless, is another benefit of the self-help industry; practices of self-help supplement and thus obscure the deficiencies of the practices of 'help' such that calls to change these are muffled.

Social relations

The construction of discourses of the personal has important implications for the way the experience of being depressed is expressed through the self's actions or practices. These will be discussed through an examination of three activities: manifestations, diversions and seeking medical help.

Looking at manifestations first, then, Lake (1987, p. 13) says:

> [depression] can take away your ability to enjoy intimacy with those you love, isolating you socially even more than usual . . . You feel you are a burden to others, so miserable that in the end you stop telling the truth about how you feel even to those who care most about you.

For Lake the experience of emotional distress can result in social withdrawal, i.e. a contravention of the ideological requisite of 'intimacy' in social institutions such as the family and networks of friends, which in turn contradicts the self's idea of personal responsibility and results in the practice of self-blame.

Goldberg (1984, p. 3) describes a paradigm of depressed behaviour using an example of an hypothetical 'bereaved mother':

> Her pining for the dead child is so severe she can neither interest herself in anything else nor get off to sleep at the end of the day . . . She loses her appetite, and so cannot bring herself to eat.

In the practice of fasting the antecedents of eating, desire and hunger, are negated. This portrayal of the neglect of personal maintenance can be interpreted as playing out a reversal of the alimentary metaphor invoked by the concept of self-regulation. Refusal to eat, social withdrawal, etc. are common examples of practices associated with being depressed. Priest (1983, p. 11) points out: 'the ultimate resort of those who feel life is completely unbearable is suicide, and this is a real risk for the severely depressed'. That is, the most serious practice enacted by people who experience being depressed is that the 'self' will attempt some act on the body aimed at discontinuing the awareness of an emotionally painful way of being. Thus, one reading of this aspect of the experience of being depressed is as resistance to the ideology and practices of self-regulation, manifested in attacks on, or neglects of, the 'self'.

A second series of practices is diversionary activities. McRae (1986, p. 45) found some comfort in music which: 'didn't dispel my sadness, but in a strange way enabled me to drift outside of myself, so that I became an observer of my own suffering'. So through the practice of listening to music, McRae's sense of self became distanced from the immediate awareness of emotional distress. Examples of other 'less laudable' diversionary practices are noted by Priest (1983, p. 23): 'Escape may come in the form of alcoholism or some other form of drug abuse.'

Finally, the practice of seeking medical help is described in Goldberg's (1984, p. 3) narrative about a bereaved mother (note that for this account Goldberg uses an emotive familial tragedy rather than circumstances, such as redundancy, with wider social causes and ramifications): 'She experiences a pervasive sense of hopelessness and despair. If her husband does not seek help, she is quite likely to kill herself.' It becomes the husband's responsibility to bridge the gap between personal and medical discourse because i) she may not be able to do it for herself, and ii) she may perform a suicidal practice. But in her autobiographical account, McRae (1986, p. 46), voices concern about the power relations between medical and personal discourse in conversation with her friend Rita:

> 'What else can my doctor do?' I asked. 'I don't want him to send me to hospital. They'd probably give me ECT [electro-convulsive therapy] which I don't want.'

McRae is afraid that if she approaches her doctor again she will be forced into a medical institution and subjected to a coercive medical practice, i.e. she imagines herself positioned within medical discourse as a powerless subject. This fear goes some way to being realized when McRae visits her doctor with Rita:

> 'I know [she needs more help],' replied the doctor, 'but there's nothing more I can do unless she breaks down. Then I can get her into hospital, where she'll be able to have ECT.' (p. 47)

Interestingly, as with Priest above, the doctor identifies the point at which he, an agent of medical discourse, can further intercede as that when McRae 'breaks down', i.e. the moment the individual is judged as no longer able to maintain a discourse of the self. This judgement may be made by: i) the individual, ii) others they interact with in a variety of discourses, such as social, familial, work, etc., and iii) (in a special case of the second category) agents of medical discourse.

Lake's emphasis on the maintenance of personal responsibility casts a different light on the decision to seek medical help:

> Some of [the steps that can be taken] ... are medical methods of dealing with depression, in the sense that you need the help of doctors to make use of them, and also in the sense that they have been developed by applying medical science and medical logic to the problem. (p. 15)

In contrast to McRae, Lake constructs the power relations between personal and medical discourse such that the individual retains personal responsibility and agency, i.e. the unitary rational subject decides whether or not to engage in further self-regulation. Also, by describing those medical services as only 'some' of the steps the self can use, Lake is confirming the power of medical discourse.

All three practices discussed above can be regarded as challenging dominant discourses of self-regulation and personal responsibility. However, paradoxically, while manifestations and diversions are pathologized, seeking medical help is presented as the apotheosis of *responsible* abdication of personal responsibility.

The dominant medical discourse defines depression in terms of physical and psychological symptoms, e.g. the APA's DSM-III-R. It follows that, in practice, depression should be 'diagnosed' or identified through the presence of these symptoms. Pitt (1993, p. vii) points out that for a GP this practice can be problematic:

> many [people] ... do not know they are depressed: they think either that they are physically or morally deficient. Alas, too often their doctors fail to make this diagnosis for them.

The occasion that permits this truth-telling is the RCP and RCGP's five-year education campaign entitled 'Defeat Depression'. By now it should be clear that the construction of 'depression' that this campaign is offering is questionable: it is partial and bolsters specific institutional practices and subject positions, such as drug treatments from GPs. Rowe (1983, p. 15) writes about the action of prescribed medication: 'Anti-depressant drugs have the effect of reversing or limiting the physiological changes that occur when a person becomes depressed.' She points out that medication alone cannot change the personal psychological qualities she argues are the cause of depression. For Rowe, the person who experiences being depressed should also receive treatment in the form of psychotherapy sessions with a clinical psychologist.

In terms of commercial discourse, however, the cost of such labour-intensive and time-consuming services, as compared to the provision of medication, is prohibitive. Both public and private medical institutions offer psychotherapeutic services to the public, but those of the public who can afford it may receive those services relatively quickly by engaging in a new financial contract with a private practice. In terms of self-regulation, individuals are classified in an explicitly structural (rather than personal) way which creates a two-tier system based on the ability to pay.

Finally, as a result of consultation during the first year of the 'Defeat Depression' campaign, the DOH, the major purveyor of governmental discourse on this matter, sent 'advice' to every GP in England and Wales. The recommendations are principally concerned with increasing the detection of depression. This practice produces further governmental pressure on medical institutions, as the proprietors and regulators of depression, to improve their services.

Before beginning my concluding comments, I should like to point out that any substantial consideration of the effects of commercial and governmental discourses, two powerful and influential social forces, could not be found in the texts examined. Once again, it is through such omissions that the personal/medical model of depression becomes dominant, legitimated by the wider social structures it leaves untheorized.

Self-help and self-regulation revisited

'What sort of a plant can he be when we don't believe a word he says?'
...
'Never you mind what sort of plant. Muddying pools. Poisoning wells, maybe. That damn sort.'
John Le Carré, *Tinker, Tailor, Soldier, Spy*

I have situated my exploration of the notions of regulation and resistance in a discourse analysis of several 'self-help' texts on the topic of 'depression'. I have suggested that the beneficiaries of this self-help industry are multiple, including authors, publishers and the State. The latter, in particular, gains much from a liberal humanist tradition that emphasizes personal responsibility and so moves attention away from larger social problems like unemployment, domestic violence, racial prejudice, etc., that form the context for much personal distress. I have argued that any particular conceptualization of 'depression' has complex implications for the person who experiences being depressed in terms of cause, treatment and cure. Through an examination of educational discourse, I have shown how authors construct their 'expert' status: a powerful subject position which enables the establishment of 'facts'. Self-regulation of individuals by the State works through this control of information and the privileging of particular 'expert' interpretations. This is particularly pronounced in the construction of the dominant medical discourse of depression as a 'psychological illness'.

Neither regulation and resistance nor self-help and self-regulation are oppositions; rather, they merge in a way indeterminable to an outside observer. They form conceptual Mobius loops which can only begin to be understood by situating oneself, for example, personally, socially or politically, on the loop. But through the complex interaction of powerful discourses, aligned randomly but in such a way as to reinforce each other, one particular viewpoint may be promoted to the detriment of all others. Thus business and governmental discourse act to promote the medical discourse's construction of 'depression' and it is the latter's informational and interpretational hegemony that must be challenged at a societal level.

Medical institutions are but one of a multiplicity of sites in which knowledges about depression are generated, e.g. personal experience (such as William Golding's *Darkness Visible*), alternative healthcare, drug companies, etc. Nor are these alternative knowledges unproblematic. While acknowledging the need to generate metaphors of experiences such as 'depression', I have demonstrated that these metaphors, by their basic function of standing in place for something else, can be damaging when we lose sight of the *unspeakable* aspects of the experiences they signify.

It would be nice if, like a magician, having illustrated some of the difficulties of the trick of defining 'depression', I could now go ahead and do it anyway – especially from my 'privileged' position as someone who identifies as experiencing depression. But that would be a very grey kind of magic and another damaging illusion. Instead I must refute simple monolithic answers and champion particular and situated complexity: 'Muddying pools . . . That damn sort.' Still, in terms of personal resistance, it might help someone experiencing being depressed to know that the cause(s) of their distress is (are) not known, to choose from interpretations of 'depression' that acknowledge their contingency, and to be able to generate personal interpretations that will be heard rather than be subsumed by some particular instantiation of medical discourse. If all this were so, perhaps (*pace* Rowe) books on depression would be more enlightening.

Robin Allwood

Appendix: Self-help books used in analysis

GOLDBERG, D. P. B. (1984) *Depression*, Edinburgh, Churchill Livingstone.
LAKE, T. (1987) *Defeating Depression*, London, Penguin Books.
McRAE, M. (1986) *A State of Depression*, London, Macmillan.
PITT, B. (1993) *Down with Gloom! or How to Defeat Depression*, London, Gaskell.
PRIEST, R. (1983) *Anxiety and Depression*, London, Martin Dunitz.
ROWE, D. (1983) *Depression: The Way Out of Your Prison*, London, Routledge & Kegan Paul.

Chapter 3

Pathologizing children:
Psychology in education and acts of government

Tom Billington

Exposition

In this chapter I argue that psychology contributes to the social regulation of children in ways, and for reasons, which usually remain unacknowledged. I consider psychology's remit in this process of regulation to be dependent on two interdependent principles: first, through adopting a medicalized, hierarchical model of symptom definition, allocation and distribution, psychology is able to locate issues of mental hygiene and thus confirm the (social) pathologization of individual children (see Foucault, 1961; Ford, Mongon and Whelan, 1982; Barton, 1989; Hollway, 1989). Second, through the exercising of a professional expertise or knowledge, individual psychologists are required to conduct (often unwittingly) this regulation of children's lives in accordance with the economic and political demands of government (Rose, 1989; Rose and Miller, 1992).

In order to explore these principles, the chapter is divided into two main parts. The first is based on a position that demands that our current understanding of psychology, children and 'special needs' be informed by an historical context. This historical context incorporates economic concepts such as the 'division of labour' and 'surplus value', concepts which were made visible during capitalism's own childhood during the eighteenth and nineteenth centuries. It is not possible here to consider these particular concepts in any detail but I need to declare that they are all, nevertheless, intrinsic to my use of the term 'market' and are otherwise active throughout the chapter.*

The second part of the chapter considers the social practices and individual 'everyday dilemmas' (Billig *et al.*, 1988) of my work as an educational psychologist, using agencies which are produced by discourses of regulation, while also looking for methods of resistance. Elsewhere in this book, authors deal more specifically with the potentials of deconstruction and discourse for

---

* Detailed consideration is given to these concepts at source in, among others, Smith, A. (orig. 1776) in Skinner, A. (Ed.) (1970) and Marx, K. (orig, 1844, 1849, 1857) in McLellan, D. (Ed.) (1977). These concepts are explored further in PhD research (as yet unfinished).

analysing issues of power and control (see also Parker and Shotter, 1990; Parker, 1992; Burman, 1994a). In this chapter, however, economic analyses are mobilized in order to consider the acts of government which live inside individual and social psychological practices within education. The two parts of the chapter are linked, and become linked with other chapters, at points of regulation and resistance.

Overall, compared with later ones, this chapter tends to emphasize the regulatory work of both psychology and the psychologist at the expense of consideration of their capacities for resistance. In searching for possible points of resistance, however, the chapter assumes a non-reductive view of power, implicitly poses the need for economic resistance at an organized, political level and works to find possibilities for personal resistance within individual, psychological practices. I conclude by suggesting that, in my work as an educational psychologist, I have found that the ideas and practices associated with discourse analysis and psychodynamic methodologies hold potentials for political resistance, both at an institutional and at a personal level. While the chapter relates to Britain and more specifically to particular forms and contexts of educational provision and 'special needs' legislation within England and Wales, the dilemmas, institutional locations and strategies should be of general relevance.

Regulation through the market

In this section I discuss the ways in which psychology interacts with market forces, pathologizing children in acts of economic regulation and distribution.

Why psychology?

Labour is the real measure of the exchangeable value of all commodities. (Adam Smith, orig. 1776, in Skinner, (Ed.) 1970, p. 133)

It is the nature of capitalized democracy that, amoeba-like, it requires ever more complex forms of 'governmentality' (Foucault, 1979a; Rose, 1989) in order to control the labours of its population. It is psychology's ability to address some of these complexities which has made it an ever-increasing part of the structures of government and an essential utility within economic life.

Psychology's utilitarian value, however, is founded on a dazzling (if usually unstated) promise, which is to define the desired 'normal' human being (who, culturally, will be adult, white, male and an owner of capital). Although not everyone yet has their own psychologist, the search for normality is being conducted by the pervasive 'psy-complex' (Ingleby, 1985; Rose, 1985) which seems to have infected all aspects of contemporary culture. It is through insidious means, such as the ones discussed throughout this book, rather than through any particular analytical or scientific brilliance, that psychology seems best able to fulfil reason's dream of controlling oneself and others (Walkerdine, 1988, after Rotman, 1980). Reason's dream, however, is one which is itself subject to powers of ownership and it is the *ownership of reason* rather than reason itself which I suggest becomes the essential site for both regulation and resistance.

Psychology has developed in order to serve not reason but the powers which seek to own reason; in the process it has assumed some of the properties of those powers it represents. An example of this is psychology's ability to generate and operate shifting, socially constructed analyses of normality and abnormality, ability and disability. Psychology is required to perform these tasks in accordance with changing economic and social demands. It achieves its authority through its alignment with *a priori* scientific enclosures of knowledge (see Rose and Miller, 1992). It is psychology's proven adaptability in continually redefining a desired normality of the human condition which makes it so attractive as a tool or social regulation, but it is an attractiveness which conveniently masks the transience of its authoritative judgements. It is only psychology's judgements which are transient, however, for its authority is fixed in firmer economic and political foundations. Psychology is allowed to represent the authoritative position only when it adheres to a particular scientific model, a model which is the product of a cultural–historical struggle.

During the last 300 years the original Latin word *scientia* (knowledge) has been absorbed by and developed within the English language until it now has a very specialized set of meanings and associations. Through the works of British empiricist philosophers such as Bacon and Hume, 'science' came to be associated with a particular method. Raymond Williams (1976, p. 278) identified a crucial moment in the battle for the word when, in 1867, science was defined as 'physical and experimental . . . to the exclusion of [the] theological and metaphysical'. Williams argued that since then, 'science' has been interchangeable, and sometimes synonymous, with 'fact, truth and reason'. In this chapter I employ the word 'science' as implying methods and practices in which the processes of 'hypothesis-generation' are unquestioned.

Once anchored in its allegiance to the authoritative, scientific position of 'fact, truth and reason', psychology is then allowed to change its judgements by generating new hypotheses in response to changing societal demands. These demands continually require different means for regulating lives, for the task of controlling economic potentials and democratic freedoms is never-ending within capitalized democracy.

Psychology – questions of economics

The West's decline in comparative wealth and industrial competitiveness has continued during the last decade in the face of a global capitalism which is busy uncovering new markets and new sources of cheap labour. The most obvious consequences within the West have been the high levels of adult male unemployment suffered in the old forms of industrial activity together with the extension of poverty, evidence of a large-scale redistribution of wealth.

These economic circumstances are challenging the traditional, essentially paternalist structures of social protection and regulation – the family and the welfare state. Many families are unable to resist the social and financial effects of this process and, increasingly, are unable to support one another. The State too is less prepared to meet economic expectations which were raised during the postwar period of welfare (Mitchell, 1974). So the same population which is now experiencing the weakening or loss of its traditional family-support system is also having to cope with a decrease in welfare provision. Increasingly in this process, children are being stripped of the fundamental economic support mechanisms, the family and the welfare state, which have been their main defences against the ultimate liberal economic dream of free competition. Governmentality through individual responsibility and entrepreneurship beckons (Rose and Miller, 1992), bringing into question the possibility of childhood itself as a discrete 'population' (Rose, 1985; Hoyles and Evans, 1989; Scarre, 1989; Cooter, 1992; Duden, 1992; Burman, 1994c).

The process in which the economic and liberal democratic expectations of people are adjusted to conform with the changing face of capital necessitates the constant regulation and redefinition of the workforce. The virulent, pathologizing forces made available by psychology continue to undertake many such acts of government in support of the market. The pathologizing forces within psychology, made available by its assumption of a medical model, are simultaneously supportive of and dependent on the democratic principles of equality of opportunity. Paradoxically, however, psychology can deny that equality of opportunity through generating discourses of abnormality and disability which are deployed within other discourses of intelligence, class, age, gender, sexuality and race. A principal, undeclared function of medicalized, social pathological methods of defining what a child should be is to refine the process of regulating access to the labour market. Discourses of abnormality and disability are economic mechanisms which contribute to the regulation of labour costs in line with the available market.

Psychology is a relatively sophisticated method of policing social and economic boundaries and in its definitions of abnormality, disability and deviance it holds the potential to justify and perform acts of social regulation and exclusion on a large scale. As various chapters in this book elaborate, psychology promises to fulfil this function not only on explicitly physical grounds (through segregating specific populations into particular institutions – the 'special' hospital, the 'special' school) but also through methods which explore more complex grounds connected to a person's inner life and which offer potentials for 'self'-regulation. This process is part of the shift in the twentieth century from physical hygiene to the complexities of mental hygiene (Rose,

1989; Urwin and Sharland, 1992). The need to consider and regulate the truths of mental life is chronicled by the explosion of social practices which revolve around psychological methods such as psychotherapy and counselling.

One of the ways in which children can be pathologized and excluded and in which (un)employability can also be regulated at an early stage is through the enclosures of knowledge which are practised by the educational psychologist. Educational psychologists broker a certain power in young lives and seek to prove their usefulness to government by regulating abnormality, disability and deviance at an early stage. Their power is based on an assumption within Western society that for many years has fuelled ideas of hope and progress: the assumption that the expansion and delivery of a medicalized knowledge of the person will of itself necessarily lead to an improvement in life circumstances. It is a responsibility of the educational psychologist to peddle this illusion that psychology, in the form of a pathologized and scientific knowledge of the (occasionally 'inner') person, works with care for the good of children who have 'special needs' or for the benefit of children who are 'at risk'.

I now argue that the actual care and the science on offer is often minimal, but the power that demands such representation is not.

Children and childhood

During the eighteenth and nineteenth centuries children and childhood in Western societies became subject to the conditions of the division of labour (Smith, 1776, in Skinner, (Ed.) 1970 and Marx 1844, 1849, 1857 in McLellan, (Ed.) 1977). A consequence of these conditions as applied specifically to children in the twentieth century is that they have become the most 'intensively governed sector of personal existence' (Rose, 1989, p. 121).

Currently in Britain, individual technologies of government (see Rose and Miller, 1992) such as developmental psychology, together with specific parliamentary legislation such as the 1993 Education Act, form and reform in order to adjust both the concept of childhood and the material circumstances of children. A purpose of these measures of government has been to identify and restrict what is feared to be the spontaneous animalism or potential for unreason within human beings (see Foucault, 1961): forces which, we are now encouraged to believe, are at their most pure, least controllable and most potent during childhood. For nearly 200 years much of the machinery of government and social regulation has been targeted at the identification and elimination of unreason. Passion and unreason are confined by acts of government and one of these confines of passion and unreason lies within the concept of childhood. It is through the definition and regulation of childhood that we can identify one of the categories of resistance against a regulation which seeks to impose itself in the name of reason.

A function of psychological practices within education has been to perform acts of government which have enabled the identification and pathologization of children whose very being is considered unreasonable: children who are allocated a social disability in whatever form, physical, mental or emotional. The success of these acts of government has to some extent depended on the daily stealth and apparent innocuousness of psychological discourses within education in order that the unreason within children's lives is made more visible. Through its ability to confirm the pathology and thus to regulate, educational psychology contributes to the assault on children's resistance to the power of reason, government and responsibility, both at a structural and at an individual level.

Special needs and the market

During the last 25 years a plethora of child legislation has reflected the tensions of changing social power relations. These changes relate to the structure of the family and the power of the individual, both parent and child (see Hoyles and Evans, 1989; Scarre, 1989; Parton, 1991; Cooter, 1992; Burman, 1994a). These changes have opened a gap in the market for a different kind of child regulation. The growth of the 'children industry', of which this chapter is inevitably a part, is evidence of the economic opportunity. Children now seem less subject to direct control by their parents and also less subject to the controls exercised by welfare provision. Instead, children are more subject to the pervasive regulation of the market. Legislative attitudes shift in order to regulate such a change regarding the minimum wage, for example, or in reducing the amounts of benefits which help to sustain discrete, traditional family units.

The continued expansion of regulation in children's lives has operated under the guise of both caring for children and also protecting their rights (e.g. the 1989 Children Act, see White, Carr and Lowe, 1990). Democratic rights of protection, however, are historically and culturally specific and current conditions require that any 'rights' are paid for by the acceptance of responsibility. The current debate on the nature of children and childhood is therefore part of the necessary process of reform and adjustment which, through the conveying of rights upon children or their parents, becomes able to apportion them responsibility. Should those social responsibilities not be assumed in the desired way, the rights are withdrawn.

This debate is both the subject and object of the market and, in regulating those underlying changes in the ways that childhood itself can be perceived, constructed and controlled, legislation has interacted with economic forces to extend the operation of the market to children. This extension has resulted in an economic boom in the children and special needs industries, stimulating a host of new technologies which strive and compete to supply our needs for information and regulation. The type of information we require about children is ever more varied, as the old questions which child psychology posed concerning the age at which children should walk, talk, read or write are now supplemented by reactivated moral questions about the age at which children 'become sexual', the age at which they can be considered 'evil' and the age at which they can be made responsible for their actions (for example in the James Bulger case: see Brookner, 1994; Dyer, 1994).

The practices which enable us to refine our ability first to define and then to adjust our perceptions of the 'normal' child (for example in psychology) are constantly reworking such questions. In tandem with government legislation, these practices of redefining childhood normality actually refine a process in which we seek to justify exclusions from particular forms of social and economic life. However, when deciding whether a child has a special need, liberal, sentimentalizing discourses related to disability act to hide the powers of the market, which are able to generate such issues of child normality.

The Warnock Report (DES, 1978) was a significant contribution to the process of child pathologization. In seeking to define children with 'special needs', Warnock was responding in part to those liberal discourses of disability which genuinely sought support for those children. Indeed, the report was an attempt to find a site of resistance against the prevailing practices in which children with particular problems were either ignored or else, if necessary, condemned to a more brutal form of segregation (see Foucault, 1961, and Rose, 1985 and 1989 for more detailed, historical explanations). The social practices which developed as a consequence of the Warnock Report, however, have themselves ultimately revealed a potential which is less than philanthropic. Under the liberal guise of providing children with extra support and (loving) care, the report contributed to a system which actually works to identify and categorize children's *ab*normality – in order that the unreasonable nature of their condition be unmasked with greater precision. Chapter 7 explores children's own accounts of their exclusion; here we focus on how the acts of exclusion from the mainstream of social life have been performed as both a purpose and a consequence of the process in which children's special needs are identified.

The rapid expansion of the social practices which permeate the whole industry of children and 'special needs' within education is an aspect of government which psychology has undertaken to police and regulate. More specifically, the professional group who were given the effective professional expertise/power to manage the definition of 'special needs' under the 1981 Education Act were educational psychologists. Their success in this enterprise, performing acts of social exclusion in such a reasonable and economic fashion, has brought them further market opportunities in the 1989 Children Act and the 1994 Code of Practice. In order to seize each new opportunity, for example in being able to contribute to definitions of children who are 'at risk', educational psychologists are brought into competition with other professionals in health and social services.

For educational psychology, the 1989 Children Act has been a considerable challenge because, in order to compete, it is having to assimilate kinds of psychology which traditionally it has been required to ignore. For example, if it is to compete in the markets of 'emotional abuse' or 'children at risk', educational psychology will have to embrace psychological practices which can provide more complex analyses of inner hygiene. However, whichever psychological paradigm, or indeed whichever profession, proves most successful in these new enterprises is largely irrelevant: the ultimate arbiter of success will not be 'good' practice, but practice which can make the most effective contribution to social regulation and government in line with the economic demands of market forces.

'Statementing' – regulation and resistance

The 'populations' within a state (see Rose, 1985; Duden, 1992) are now so numerous that social regulation demands complex properties of transportability, metamorphosis and self-generation. The survival of capitalized democracy is achieved, in part, through its ability to generate such new mechanisms which can service the changing demands of mass (economic) regulation. Enterprises of government and regulation have sought to own for themselves the Enlightenment concepts of reason and progress (see Foucault, 1961; Walkerdine, 1988; Rose, 1989). One of the appeals of capitalized democracy lies in its promise of less overt forms of social coercion made possible through science and reason. It offers these while still being able to protect the interests of economic power.

Such refinements of government over the lives of children and their families have occurred at an increasing pace since Warnock. These refinements have been achieved, in part, through the activity of three interlinked processes: first, through the operation of the market; second, through psychological discourses which are rooted within social practices; and third, through a series of legislative measures. The most significant pieces of recent legislation have been the Education Acts of 1981 and 1993, and the Children Act of 1989.

A most important consequence of these measures is the extension of legalism (Parton, 1991) within the process of child measurement and regulation. This process of child assessment has been named 'formal assessment', but it is often known as 'statementing'. This process has been refined further by the Code of Practice (DFE, 1994) which relates to the 'identification and assessment of children with special educational needs'. There exists a whole arena for social practices through which the government of children and their families can be exercised. These 'formal' procedures can involve many different participants, from teachers and headteachers to doctors and health workers, from local education administrators and welfare officers to the police and social workers, and from educational and clinical psychologists to parents and children. This huge enterprise in the social regulation of children was instigated partially under the guise of liberal, individualist discourses such as 'individual potentials', 'the needs of the individual' and 'individual rights', but it was also instigated by an economic need to rationalize the allocation of resources.

I should make clear, however, that this analysis does not deny that there can be significant benefits for many of the children and families (and also schools) who go through the 'statementing' process, through the allocation of extra resources, for example. A wide variety of specialist help can be accessed, medical help such as speech therapy or physiotherapy, individual adult care for children who have a physical disability, or further educational resources such as computers or teaching support, all of which can bring positive material benefits to individual children and their families. These benefits form part of the process of resistance and fuel dilemmas of individual experience of psychological practices (Billig *et al.*, 1988). Discourses of 'help' and 'need', and all of the social practices surrounding 'statementing', despite their capacity to attract individual benefits and notwithstanding the undoubted personal commitment of individual practitioners, are resistances against the fundamental, regulatory potentials for social exclusion within the assessment process.

It is in this way that regulation and resistance combine to work and govern together through complex social practices. The visibility of either the regulation or the resistance will, however, depend largely on the position of the individual participants within the system of power relations (Henriques *et al.*, 1984; Hollway, 1989; Parker and Shotter, 1990; Parker, 1992).

Looking to resist

Educational psychologists owe their continuing survival as professionals to their ability to hold and service the dilemmas which are sites of regulation and resistance. In order to perform their professional roles and activities, educational psychologists need to be able to move easily from regulation to resistance and vice versa. This fluidity is made possible by the variability of the power which is vested in the title and role of 'educational psychologist' (Billington, 1995). The unfixed, rather vague nature of educational psychology allows the individual practitioner to move between and make contact with the various positions of the other participants in a series of changing power relations. Inside the process, each psychologist is able to perform less obviously coercive acts of government in the name of science, reason and welfare.

The potentials for resistance within those liberal discourses of helping the 'needy', etc. are used by the psychologist who in the process will often claim child advocacy in order to fulfil such tasks. On the other hand, however, the demand for psychologists to perform regulatory acts of exclusion and enforcement are also often enacted through claiming that same position of child advocacy. This position is not always claimed, but such examples highlight the power of psychologists and their expertise, either to be static or fluid, to regulate, or else to resist in a complex web of power relations. The structured role of the educational psychologist within the assessment process is one designed to hold these dilemmas as an act of government. In the process, individual psychologists provide a site for the fundamental but often elusive opposition of regulation and resistance which is the subject of this book.

Whose need?

The bulk of referrals to educational psychologists have traditionally emanated from schools, supposedly on behalf of the child. So what is it that schools seek to achieve from the referral? Why do schools refer children to psychology? My own experience reflects that of Ford *et al.* (1982) who found that schools often refer children to the psychologist in order to meet their own needs rather than to meet the needs of the child. This is part of a process, now refined further by the Code of Practice (DFE, 1994), which can lead to material rewards through acts of pathologization.

The government's policy of Local Management of Schools (LMS) has demanded that schools now operate according to a fixed budget which is delegated directly to them. In the past, schools have been financed through the Local Education Authority (LEA) and that method of financing often enabled schools to access various forms of extra funding or further resources. Local Management of Schools has, effectively, closed down that access and one of the only possibilities remaining for a school to gain extra resources is through the special educational needs budget, a portion of which has remained in the control of the Local Education Authority.

Schools are often attracted by the process of formal assessment of special educational needs because of its potential rewards. One of its rewards can be the allocation of extra resources from that Local Education Authority special educational needs budget in order to address the needs of the child within the school. Should this resource not meet the school's needs, however, they can still benefit from the assessment process through, in some cases, a removal from the school altogether of the child seen as the problem (see also Marks, Chapter 7). Deals are struck all the time. Sometimes children are only allowed to remain in the referring school on the promise of an extra resource or else they are removed from the school because of the denial of that resource.

The legislation has achieved its impact on the education system through linking economic potentials directly to a 'statement' which schools are keen to access. In the assessment process, schools often see the educational psychologist as holding the key to these resources as a 'gatekeeper', for their professional expertise in describing a 'special need' is vital within the legal framework. Schools therefore often exert pressure on the psychologists to diagnose a child's 'need' in order to gain an extra resource from which they will be the prime beneficiary. A recurring dilemma for the individual psychologist is that their employers, the Local Education Authority, often pressurize them *not* to ascribe a 'special need' because of the finite nature of their available resources.

In the (social, medicalized) pathologization of children which has become embedded within 'special needs', therefore, the question of 'whose need is being addressed?' itself needs to be raised. This question provides a site for analysing the power relations and investments at stake and therefore holds the potential for the organization of resistance. Psychologists often exercise considerable individual resolve within the process of allocating 'need', particularly if they use their *powers* of judgement upon a child in ways which do not satisfy the school's economic demands. In such instances, a pressure to actually remove the child can build up in the school, a pressure which appears irresistible. Schools can begin to amass the evidence to justify that removal, while the child can suffer considerable distress at the realization that the school's (psychological) commitment to them has been severed. The effects of this on the child could be seen as akin to 'separation anxiety' (Freud, 1986; Klein, 1988; Winnicott, 1971, 1986). Such an analysis provides evidence of the way in which psychology can, at the same point, provide a site both for regulation *and* resistance; the selection of one at the expense of the other can rest with the individual psychologist.

At the realization of the predicated consequences for such a child, where the psychologist has not complied with the school's wishes, the psychologist has to decide whether to confirm the school's own pathologization of the child, whether to assert their own, or whether to deny the pathologization altogether. These decisions make visible personal choices between regulation and resistance. A decision to resist then demands a further decision as to where the resistance should be placed: within the school or within a new situation.

Which child?

It is schools, therefore, who often have both the need and the power to conduct the initial act of pathologization on children by employing psychological discourses. But which children do they select for 'treatment'? The process in which schools identify a child as needing a psychological referral is itself evidence that the pathologization of the child has already been started by the school and often it is only a confirmation of a diagnosis which is sought. Schools usually organize the evidence for their pathologization around three sets of criteria: 'learning', 'behavioural' and 'medical'. This chapter does not claim any statistical 'truths', neither does it make uncontestable claims for the statistical generalizability of the following figures. Also, it should be noted that, within these figures I am circulating traditional forms of categorization and possible segregation. Nevertheless, it is informative to note that the referrals I received during the two-month period in which I first drafted this chapter (November and December 1993) fell into this pattern:

Tom Billington

| | Type of school | | | |
| | Primary | | Secondary | |
	Boy	Girl	Boy	Girl
Reason for referral				
Statutory reassessment	5	2	5	–
New referrals				
'learning difficulties'	1	5	–	–
'behaviour problems'	13	–	–	3
'medical problems'	1	2	–	–

In a brief unscrambling of those figures several points seem obvious. I was asked to see more boys than girls, asked to see more children with behavioural difficulties than for any other category and asked to see more primary school children than secondary. The overwhelming number of children I saw came from homes which were far from affluent. The only child from a 'middle-class' home who was referred within the 'behaviour' category was the subject of an interesting dispute – perhaps itself an example of the ways in which class privilege can (attempt to) ward off the greater social stigmatization of 'maladjustment' – as the parents actually saw the problem as one of 'learning' rather than 'personality difficulties'.

'Behaviour' is the largest category. Boys in secondary schools were often not referred, however, unless they were the subjects of statutory reassessments (usually of previously allocated resources). Many teenaged boys whose behaviour is 'difficult' have usually already been excluded from mainstream school and put into some other kind of institution, or else if they are still in mainstream education such boys are unwanted within the school and their educational potentials are ignored. Schools and service practices regard psychological 'help' to be a waste of time for these boys and at best any involvement would be in response to a demand for input which feels punitive rather than therapeutic. Schools usually have other ways of removing such pupils without recourse to specific psychological expertise (again, see Marks, Chapter 7).

Teenaged girls whose behaviour is creating difficulties can pose problems for their schools because, unlike the boys, they are less likely to have been identified by the exclusion process during their primary years (see also Davies, 1984). Often there is no alternative punitive placement available and recently, therefore, pressures within schools to exclude girls seem to be mounting. But, partly because there is no other provision and partly by virtue of the gender stereotyping structured within 'talking cures', schools do seem more likely to consider a more therapeutic involvement for girls rather than for boys. The therapeutic mode is in any case usually denied by psychologists on the grounds of insufficient time and resources. Within that denial, however, there often seem to live thinly veiled suspicions that forms of counselling are either ineffective or else too soft on the individual subject, while more psychotherapeutic methods are regarded as being in some way radical, subversive or not real 'scientific' psychology (see Winnicott, 1986).

In primary schools, girls' behaviour sometimes seems almost invisible (Kelly, 1988; Billington, 1993) and it is boys who have been brought to my attention in considerable numbers. Cultural gender discourses abound in the primary schools, for example, obvious ones such as 'boys are active' and 'girls need protecting'. It is becoming possible to see points at which the sympathetic, amused 'aah' factor relating to little boys' naughty behaviour (employing discourses such as 'boys will be boys') suddenly switches into the fear of both the same boys and their behaviour. It is at about the time of this 'switch' that the power of the educational psychologist can often be sought, for the otherwise unbridled (sexual) energies (or passion) of such boys constitute a threat to reason and order (Walkerdine, 1981, 1990). In this way the school announces the pathology and thus begins the social, economic *and* psychological processes of severance and exclusion.

In practice, it has been possible for me to resist this process on behalf of a child, particularly where there are individuals within the school who are also prepared to resist the dominant pressures. There are individual schools and teachers who, while aware of their regulatory function, have gone to considerable lengths to resist the seeming inevitability of the removal process. Often, however, where there is no possibility of a collective resistance, individual resistance on behalf of the child can be either futile, untenable or unbearable for any adult and also, perhaps, for the child. The power of regulation has eyes only for impersonal resistances to its own power and, while experienced by the recipients at an individual level, possibilities for asserting their own power can often be denied by the individual psychologist. For there are dangers that, in choosing to exercise their power by offering resistance, an individual psychologist may well be attributed with the same characteristics of deviance previously attributed to the child.

Measuring, pathologizing and 'treating' children

The practices of psychological expertise can be confined by the pathologies which the schools choose to diagnose in the original referral. The children who have medical difficulties tend to be considered least problematic for their pathology, and the expectations of treatment for them, are currently understood as lying outside the expertise of both schools and psychologists. A common treatment for children who are diagnosed as having behaviour difficulties is the prescription by the psychologist of a behaviour-modification programme, while children with learning difficulties are typically given forms of psychometric assessment followed by a structured learning programme.

In order to fulfil its customary obligations of social regulation and pathologization, psychology within education has, with only token exceptions, adopted the principles and practices of an extreme positivism. In practice, the principal task of the educational psychologist has been to measure children, their abilities, their attainments and their behaviours. The purpose of these activities has been to identify disability or deviance in any of its forms – physical, mental or emotional – on behalf of the State and in order to facilitate the processes of economic regulation.

While discourses of individual needs are essential to the practices of educational psychology, the formal assessment procedures ('statementing') both generate and respond to discourses and social practices of special needs which are, in effect, audits of individual lives. The most economically efficient means of performing these acts of accounting is through measurement, stat(e)istics, the 'science of state' (Rose, 1989). Measurement is a core activity for educational psychologists and, together with the application of linear cause-and-effect models to most situations, is one which is established in professional training. In order to conduct the most efficient, cost-effective means of social analysis and regulation, educational psychology has adopted simplistic models of psychological practice in which children's identities can be reduced to the smallest number of features possible in the shortest time available. Indeed, educational and psychological practices can often operate in ways which deny their subjects any identity whatsoever.

It is economic pressures which demand that the individual psychologist should 'deal (quickly) with' the referred children. The sheer volume of children who are pathologized by their schools has a significant effect on the kind of psychology which is permitted – the kind of lives which can be accepted – for such large numbers demand that a reductionist psychology is imposed on and attributed to children and their families. Simplistic analyses are preferred, together with analyses which deftly avoid more liberal, humanist discourses of individual rights and feelings.

The exclusive application of linear, hypothesis-forming-and-testing models of psychological practice conjures the illusion that the psychologist is invisible and liberal notions of reflexivity, analyses of the processes of hypothesis-generation, or the employment of psychodynamic paradigms, are all regarded as radical and as potential threats to the regulation. Time is so limited within the demanded model that only the child's behaviour can be seen. Through such individualizing and through concentration on 'problem-focused' practices, not only is their failure made likely but the child can also be made to confirm their own pathology.

In using acts of measurement which operate under the aegis of science and reason, the process of regulation meets with oppositions from a whole range of liberal discourses concerning children's rights (for example the right to moral choices and the right to feelings) which become enmeshed in a complex web. In practice, however, any rights to be viewed as an individual are accorded to children in only two circumstances: either because they are a member of a higher social order, or because of the retrospective attribution of responsibilities in the event of a social misdemeanour.

The psychometric test has long been the main weapon in the psychologist's armoury against children who are diagnosed as possessing 'learning difficulties' (see Rose, 1985, for an historical account of the struggle between medicine and psychology for control of this expertise). Its value lies in its ability to reduce any individual to a single figure, an offer which has been too good to refuse. Psychometrics have proved to be an effective weapon in the battery of assessment techniques which are used to regulate and pathologize children. It is significant that, before and during my training as an educational psychologist, I always maintained that I would never use any 'tests'. I now make considerable use of them, however, justifying their use as weapons of resistance, to reflect back as counter-discourses and challenge the contest that the technologies created.

For example, I have used tests of 'learning ability' with those young boys who were referred to me for having behaviour problems. In such cases, the tests have initially provided the basis for a good working relationship between myself and the child. Undoubtedly, I occupy the position of structural power, but in trying to make the actual performance of the tests one of choice as well as one of regulation, it feels, paradoxically, as though a 'potential space' (Winnicott, 1971) has been created in which the child and myself can play and build a relationship. In this way I can commit myself to the child at a more individual level.

Children are often surprised when they realize that the school's pathologization of them, which exists in their negative relationship, is not central in our relationship. However, neither are the children asked for an unreasonable trust, for they are not asked to suspend their knowledge that my presence has been requested by the school to serve the school's interests (as one colleague remarked, 'children don't refer themselves'). The importance of the approach is that it provides a site for resistance, enabling me to challenge the school's pathology while, through reflexive means, being able to challenge and resist any subsequent attempts to impose a pathology of my own on to the individual child.

Under such conditions, without exception, all the children I tested scored at least what psychometricians would describe as 'within the expected range'. Indeed, several of them scored very high marks. Now these were all children who were poor academic achievers within school and who were seen as problems by the school because of their behaviour. Their test scores therefore became a point of resistance as I was able to employ the authority vested in my professional role on behalf of the child, invoking the powers of science and reason in order to resist and refute the school's pathology. In such a way, I was trying to shift the individuals within the school away from seeing a pathologized behaviour in order that they might be able to employ different analyses.

In effect, I was using the power of the methods which are normally applied in the pathologization of 'learning difficulties' to resist the pathologization of behaviour. Conversely, I would argue that it may be possible to use alternative paradigms to resist the pathologization of 'learning difficulties' (Bettelheim and Zehan, 1982; Klein, 1988, 1989; Sinason, 1992). Significantly, however, attempts to use psychodynamic language as a site for resistance have themselves met with resistance. Alternative, psycho-dynamically-based analyses of children's learning have been resisted, I would suggest, because of their potential both to demand the engagement of all the participants and to avoid the pathologization of the specified individuals (Henriques *et al.*, 1984; Hollway, 1989).

All psychological practices produce their own political problems and in using any methods for the purposes of resistance I am also contributing to the process of regulation. However, such methods reveal points of contestation and power, of meaning and interpretation (Hollway, 1989; Parker, 1992) at which the potential for regulation and resistance becomes analysable. In prac-tice, the 'natural', 'desired' alternative to my chosen strategy would be to accept the school's pathologization of behaviour difficulties and then impose behaviour modification techniques, methods which are unable to mask the primitivism of their regulatory intent. Such techniques are often applied in order that the individual cannot be seen and the object of intervention is to relate a behaviour to the demands of a presenting authority. So it is only the effects of the behaviour which are important both to the school and to the psychologist, for the causes of those effects, according to the simplistic theory of the social offered by behaviourist models, are considered to reside in the immediate, physical circumstances.

This suppression of socioeconomic circumstances is over-determined by another factor, for the workings of the unconscious are not explored by the psychologist, both on ideological grounds and also because the attribution of a complex inner life to children and other 'clients' would be deemed unaccept-able. Behaviour modification is preferred, as just one more step in the process of assessing whether a child may eventually become amenable to social con-trol. If the 'programme' works, fine. If not, the child's failure will provide justification for their ultimate removal not only from the school, but subse-quently from other strata of social activity. By such means, behaviour modifi-cation techniques also allow the school or psychologist to allocate a pathology which in the process enables them to rationalize their own refusal to engage with the child at an individual level. While the teachers and psychologists have the power to justify their actions as reason itself, the effects of their pathologization may actually live in the child's individual experience. It is in such ways that teachers and psychologists seek to avoid the individual, experi-ential consequences of their own regulatory actions.

Just as the technology of testing can be used to work against the structures of classification and segregation they were devised to police, I would argue that psychodynamic methods of working might more readily address the in-equality of (interpersonal) power relations. Psychodynamic approaches, while also complicit in producing docile, self-regulating individuals, at least have the potential to demand the experiential presence of the individual psychologist, another authority figure. Such methods can work to expose rather than repress both the reality and the subjectivity of the psychologist's acts of coercion. The employment of such 'radical' paradigms can uncover the traces of regulation at an individual level and may yet offer opportunities for individual and institutional resistance.

Conclusions

To sum up, the effects of many psychological practices and discourses within education are:

1 to pathologize and to regulate;
2 to deny individuality to the recipients of practices;
3 to define children and their families within narrow, value-laden limits;
4 to deny the effects on the practitioner of both their subjectivity and their structured position;
5 to restrict the allocation of resources;
6 to employ superficial, simplistic and oppressive working practices;
7 to reject unconscious processes as a legitimate concern of practice;
8 to allow or deny access both to a psychologist and to particular psychological practices according to social class, gender and race (see also Billington, 1995).

This chapter has tried to expose some of the ways in which psychological practices are (economic) acts of government. Psychology performs these acts of government through procedures of regulation and pathologization which infect our practices so insidiously that it is difficult to make them visible. The emphasis has been on exposing those connections, rather than to stress that regulation is necessarily wrong. This is because to question either the necessity to regulate or the rights of government to participate in that regulation is beyond the remit of this chapter, although these are political issues that clearly arise from this analysis.

The purpose of emphasizing the regulatory and pathologizing functions of psychology in this chapter has been in order to expose the ways in which, too often, psychologists are drawn by the power of government into practices which require them to surrender their science to the demands of that governmental power. It is suggested that psychology needs to work hard to understand its own economic, regulatory and pathologizing functions so that it can leave the more obvious acts of government to more obvious means of government and begin to find its own ethical science.

On a personal level, resisting these regulatory and pathologizing tendencies which are demanded by a professional role can exact a considerable toll.

For what purpose, when it feels as though that resistance merely feeds the need and sharpens the ability to regulate? The fundamental demand made of me as an educational psychologist seems to be that I disguise myself in order to confront and undermine individual lives with the power of society's desire to regulate them. The difficulty of practice is compounded by the dilemma posed by the liberal discourses of special needs, for current psychological practices can indeed benefit individual lives. In order to improve its potential to benefit those individual lives, however, psychology should find the means of resisting the pathologizing tendency which is demanded by the powers of government. I believe that non-oppressive, psychological practices can find a site for potential resistance in the collective knowledge and practices which are to be found in psychodynamic approaches:

> The very nub of [Freud's] work was the elimination of an absolute difference between abnormality and normality. (Mitchell, 1974, p. 11)

I suggest that psychodynamic approaches possess various theoretical and ethical possibilities for working with people in ways which can resist both the concept of an absolute normality and also the demands to pathologize – although, admittedly, current practices do not always make use of that potential.

Whichever the paradigm, however, behavioural, psychometric or psychodynamic, I have argued in this chapter that it is the meanings and values of the measures of pathologization in supporting particular acts of government, rather than specifically the act of measurement itself, which is necessarily so abhorrent about the ways in which customary psychological practices have infected children and education. It is these meanings and values which can also be addressed by the turn to discourse (Billington, 1995). Discourse analytic methods can provide sites for the analysis of and therefore the subsequent resistance against such meanings and values, together with the power relations on which they feed.

The pathologization of children and childhood which has been made available through psychology is, primarily, a method of imposing the government and power of social and economic demands under a guise of science and reason. A psychology which draws on both discourse analytic and psychodynamic principles might yet hold potentials for resisting the pathologizing tendency. In order to realize these potentials and in the market 'trade-off' between regulation and resistance, it will be important for such methods neither to reject science and reason, nor to deny economic and political analyses, but rather to compete more strongly for their ownership.

Chapter 4

Feminist therapy and its discontents

Colleen Heenan

Feminism and psychotherapy

For many years, feminism and psychotherapy have had an uneasy, at times even hostile relationship. Classic feminist texts such as Phyllis Chesler's *Women and Madness* (1972), highlighted the gender bias of psychiatry. This demonstrated not only how its practice reproduced popular narratives of women, but also revealed that, in their aims to normalize, male practitioners sometimes even sexually abused their female clients. Further, Broverman *et al.*'s (1970) classic paper, 'Sex-role stereotypes and clinical judgements of mental health' made it clear that psychology's criteria for 'normal' mental health were clearly biased towards characteristics deemed to be 'masculine'. There seemed little doubt in the minds of most feminists that, far from being the 'caring' professions, these disciplines represented a danger to women's mental health. This belief is encapsulated in radical feminists like Mary Daly's (1979) reading of the word 'therapist', as 'the rapist'.

However, while radical lesbian feminists such as Kitzinger and Perkins (1993) still see psychotherapy and feminism as an anathema, many other feminists believe psychotherapeutic, especially psychoanalytic, theory affords feminists the possibility of more fully understanding the ways in which not only is 'the personal political' but also how the 'political *becomes* personal'. For instance, in 1976 Jean Baker Miller explicated the ways in which psychoanalytic theory was dominated by patriarchal discourses which privileged notions of the unitary, rational (male) subject, thus devaluing characteristics deemed to be feminine. This allowed women not only to reclaim but to celebrate their 'otherness' to men. Other psychotherapists such as Luise Eichenbaum and Susie Orbach (1982, 1983, 1987) drew on psychoanalytic object relations theory to develop a feminist psychoanalytic analysis of the shaping of gender and personality. Along with Dinnerstein (1976) and Chodorow (1978, 1989), they deconstructed the ways in which gendered subjectivities are constructed within and reproduced by (heterosexual) families and relationships.

This attention to deconstructing the interrelationship between the internal, psychological and external, social world is one way in which feminist psychotherapy's concerns with the 'project of the self' mirrors

Colleen Heenan

poststructuralist concerns with the 'project of subjectivities'. Authors like Elshtain (1982) argue that a thorough grasp of concepts relating to the unconscious could promote an epistemological shift from a dualistic model of mind to a more varied examination of its shifting and contradictory nature. Feminist post-structuralists such as Weedon (1987) suggest that psychoanalytic theory has the potential to contribute towards understanding the postmodern subject, although she sees the work of the psychoanalytic 'French feminists' such as Cixous, Irigaray and Kristeva, as offering a more thoroughly deconstructive approach than that of the feminist object relations theorists, Eichenbaum and Orbach, and Chodorow.

In this chapter, I explore the dynamic relationship between feminism, object relations therapy and post-structuralist theory. Using a feminist Foucauldian discourse analysis, I study excerpts from a clinical supervision of a feminist psychodynamic psychotherapy group for women with eating disorders. Examining the ongoing development of thought within and between feminism and psychotherapy in this context illustrates some of the tensions inherent within feminist psychoanalytic psychotherapy. Being resistive to the normalizing practices of conventional psychotherapy does not in itself mean feminist psychotherapy can escape from being regulatory. Feminist post-structuralists like Flax (1990, 1993) highlight how, in their attempts to understand subjectivity, both feminists and psychoanalysts have not theorized how *they* are constrained by their discursive underpinnings. This has resulted in them imposing their own 'grand narratives', specifically about contemporary Western, white, heterosexual middle-class 'woman', on *all* women.

In order to set the scene, I first locate myself in relation not just to my subject matter, but to the themes within the book as a whole. Next, I briefly describe the theory and practice of feminist object relations psychotherapy. Moving on to critique these models from a feminist post-structuralist perspective, I also indicate the links between feminist object relations theory and post-structuralism, especially in relation to language and deconstruction. Interwoven within this I discursively explore a feminist psychotherapy supervision. While this demonstrates the tensions between feminism and psychoanalysis, it also indicates how they contribute to one another. This extends understanding of the complex interrelationship between private and public, personal and political, so much the focus of post-structuralist thinking.

The 'I' within the 'we'

Feminist research has an enduring commitment to a reflexive paradigm (Stanley and Wise, 1983, 1993; Wilkinson, 1988). Just as the researcher needs to locate herself in relation to her research, so I need to locate myself in relation to my topic and my chapter to the book as a whole. Like my co-authors, I approach the subjects under consideration from multiple positions. As a feminist psychoanalytic psychotherapist, I have a commitment to trying

56

to both understand and change the problematic and seemingly enduring nature of contemporary Western women's subjective experiences. As a feminist, I am well aware of the ways in which epistemological and structural inequalities serve to define and exclude many women. As a woman, I have experienced some of the ways in which these inequalities are mirrored in personal relationships, not just between men and women but also between different women.

As a psychotherapist, I work with clients who are attempting to understand the interrelationship between the ways in which they are socially, culturally, historically and personally positioned in relation to others and themselves. However, these are not intellectual exercises wherein parts of self 'float like signifiers and signified' (Flax, 1990) but are very immediate bodily and emotional experiences and, clearly, the focus of therapy is mainly on clients' feelings about these issues. Chapter 2 made this point in relation to experiences of depression. At the same time, it is impossible to separate our emotional exploration from its social context as the process of therapy is thoroughly *intersubjective*, focusing 'on the interplay between the differently organised subjective worlds of the observer and the observed' (Stolorow, Brandchaft and Atwood, 1992). Further, my work with women who have eating disorders particularly highlights the socially constructed nature not only of the conscious but also the unconscious processes which act on the body, such that it becomes the site of both regulation and resistance (Heenan, 1995b). In turn, the very boundaries of our contractual relationship serve as a constant reminder of the socially constructed nature of psychotherapy.

Feminist psychotherapy both informs and reflects the modern industrialized context in which it developed. Its discursive and reflexive aspects in some respects closely ally it with postmodern concerns to understand the construction and reproduction of subjectivities. It could also be described as thoroughly postmodern in the discursive way it draws on the semantic manner of language in its desire to understand the relational nature of 'the meaning of meaning' (Frosh, 1989). Moreover, feminist psychoanalytic psychotherapy's acceptance of unconscious processes means it also focuses on the active way in which discourses are not only constructed *internally* but are also reproduced within the gendered intersubjective field of psychotherapy practice and other social relations. While Chapter 7 demonstrates the gendered nature of the exclusion process in schools, this chapter focuses on the dynamics of a feminist clinical supervision in order to deconstruct some aspects of feminist psychotherapy.

The act of researching and writing about this topic offers similar parallels. In deconstructing my topic, I am also constructing it. In taking up particular positions, I also repress some oppositions. In writing the chapter as 'I', I reveal my ongoing struggle with these issues, a struggle which is at one and the same time my own and a part of a wider concern located within the book and its audience. Like feminist psychotherapy, it is a dynamic and discursive process.

Colleen Heenan

Feminist object relations: theory and therapy

Feminist object relations theorists could be described as initiating the beginnings of what would now be termed a feminist *Foucauldian* analysis of the gendered characteristics of the internalized panopticon (Bartky, 1988). Like feminist post-structuralists, feminist psychoanalytic object relations theorists are concerned to understand the intersubjective field in which subjectivities are constructed, in particular gendered subjectivities. They attempt to articulate and understand the nuances of the resistive and regulatory aspects of 'women's problems' by adopting discursive critiques of the ways in which women draw on the available gendered discourses of femininity (Hollway, 1989), mental health and distress in order to express themselves; at the same time, adopting this stance acts to challenge the boundaries of these discourses. Using psychoanalysis they address unconscious motives. Political analysis is interwoven within this framework in order to conceptualize how a seemingly 'maladaptive' response functions to create some scope for freedom within constitutions of marginalization and oppression.

Object relations theory suggests that the construction of individual subjectivity is simultaneously affected by, as well as mirroring, social relations. It argues that symbols of self and others (objects) are introjected on an unconscious level, affording the possibility of *intra*-psychic relations within and between parts of self, as well as *inter*-psychic relations with others. Its focus on relational aspects of psychological development, especially the relationship between infant and mother, contrasts with Freud's emphasis on the sexual body and self. However, by drawing attention to the ways in which the material dimensions of power interact with emotional relations of power, feminist object relations theorists explicated the influence of social constructions of gender on internal 'objects'. For instance, Chodorow (1978) argued that the construction of male identity is premised on differentiating from women, especially from mothers, in order to deal with infantile fears of dependency on these powerful and female figures.

Further, Eichenbaum and Orbach (1983) emphasize the factors which contribute to the problematic nature of women's relationships with each other, especially between mothers and daughters. They suggest that within the current contexts of social exclusion and marginalization, mothers may be particularly unable and even unwilling to meet their daughters' needs. Highlighting the fragmented and narrowly defined images of women which prevail in contemporary Western society, these authors explore the tensions which may arise for mothers in raising daughters to take up quite constrained social positions. In particular, they make clear the ways in which women are encouraged to develop and maintain fluid psychological and physical boundaries, which they term 'emotional antennae', in order to be available to nurture others. This notion is an extension of Winnicott's concept of 'mirroring', whereby mothers are seen to participate in the construction of infants' selves by accurately reflecting their needs (Ernst, 1987).[1] Chapter 8 highlights ways in which parenting is discursively constructed.

In addition to theory, Eichenbaum and Orbach, as well as Ernst and Maguire (1987), also discuss the *practice* of feminist object relations therapy. This requires that the therapist explores not only how the client's inner world is permeated by social representations of self and other, but also how the client projects her inner world on to the outer. The intersubjective field of the therapeutic relationship provides an integral means for constructing and pursuing this process. What is specific to this is

> its concern to understand internal and external reality together. It does this in a way that recognises how external reality forms and oppresses women, at the same time as understanding the autonomy and powerfulness of internal reality. It relates inner and outer reality within a total perspective as well as keeping them separate and distinct. (Ryan, 1983, p. 9)

Eichenbaum and Orbach propose that a feminist psychoanalytic perspective enables the therapist to offer her client 'an interpretation that speaks to the full meaning of an individual woman's experience, reflects an understanding of the ways in which the material world creates individual personality, symptomatology, defence structures and so on' (1987, p. 50).

Feminist therapeutic deconstructions of depression or eating disorders problematize the way in which gendered behaviour is regulated through the promotion of notions of individual pathology (Orbach, 1978, 1986; Nairn, 1982; Lawrence, 1987). For instance, physical and psychological 'symptoms' may be manifestations of the struggles some women experience in negotiating and changing their inner and outer worlds. Some symptoms of distress such as depression, poor self-image, difficulties related to food and weight or confused feelings about expressing their sexuality are mainly experienced – or reported as experienced – by women. At the same time, some of these more covert psychological manifestations of unhappiness appear to reproduce the more passive aspects of women's gendered selves rather than being overtly challenging of their oppression. Ryan (1983, p. 16) suggests that the 'containing, exhausting, and stupefying characteristics of depression typify the feelings of powerlessness and lack of control which many women experience'.

Deconstructing the problems which women present in therapy enables us to see these as more than an individual's inability to cope with her life. Symptoms could also be interpreted as unconscious expressions of women's resistance to their experience of living in a patriarchal society. Thus, rather than describing a woman as sexually 'frigid' and thus encouraging her to feel better about having sex, a feminist therapist might explore her client's feelings about whether or not she may feel oppressed by sexual – and other – expectations her partner may have of her. If this is a heterosexual relationship, one feminist interpretation might be that this woman 'won't be fucked around'.

However, adopting a pathological career offers a form of resistance in that a depressed woman or an agoraphobic woman is often unable to carry on with, say, domestic responsibilities. Women who starve themselves, binge and vomit or eat compulsively can be understood not simply as 'victims' of media hype but as challenging social norms by being very, very good by dieting to extremes; by defying the sanction against women having an appetite, or by being more than 'little women'.

Discourse analysis and feminist psychotherapy

Feminism, psychoanalysis and post-structuralism share a commitment to semantic principles and deconstructive understanding. Frosh (1989) describes Freud's belief in the way that 'language both expresses the symbolism of the unconscious and is the means of unravelling it. It therefore embodies subjective experience but also provides a route to the source of that experience – the construction of subjectivity itself' (p. 136). Language learning and use is a thoroughly interpersonal affair in which meaning is given and received, negotiated and understood *through* relationships, from infancy to adulthood. Feminists such as Spender (1980) have demonstrated ways in which language is '*man*made', while Daly (1979) has proposed '*woman*made' alternatives. Analysing discourse is one deconstructive tool adopted by post-structuralist feminists (Weedon, 1987; Burman, 1991a, 1995). At the same time, contemporary feminists such as Hollway (1989) have incorporated psychoanalytic concepts within their discourse analytic models. Gavey (1989, p. 45) suggests it offers a methodology 'consistent with a feminist post-structuralist perspective'; that is, it offers a tool for exploring how meaning is *constituted by*, rather than *reflected in*, language.

Exploration in psychotherapy occurs through and by means of language. Discourse analysis is akin to psychotherapy, especially psychoanalytic psychotherapy wherein:

> therapy centers [sic] on meaning, and language is its medium. Therapy is an oral mode, and narratives, proverbs, metaphors, and interpretations are its substance. The metaphorical language used in therapy to represent the world is a way to try to comprehend partially what cannot be comprehended totally. (Hare-Mustin and Maracek, 1990, p. 47)

Thus, while discourse analysis, as linked with post-structuralism, mirrors psychoanalysis's interest in the construction of subjectivities, it simultaneously operates to deconstruct it.

Discourse analysis also provides a useful means of 'listening on a different level' to clinical material. It is both similar to and yet contrasts with a psycho-analytic approach. Working within a psychoanalytic framework requires that the therapist develops and incorporates a reflexive way of listening and relating to her clients; that is, she must adopt multiple positions in relation to the client, to the client's and her own conscious material and unconscious communications. However, as with any psychotherapy, an essential part of the practice of feminist psychoanalytic psychotherapy includes clinical supervision and discussion with other more experienced feminist psychoana-lytic psychotherapists. Supervision involves a retrospective analysis of client material with the clinical supervisor temporarily adopting the position of offering a meta-analysis of not only the client–therapist relationship but also the supervisor–therapist relationship. The aim of this is to enable the practi-tioner to develop an active and proactive 'internal supervisor' (Casement, 1985, 1990).

For the feminist psychotherapist, clinical supervision is particularly im-portant in that most current psychotherapy training is dominated by fairly conservative practitioners who adhere to conventional models of development which fail to critique dominant discourses of gender or sexual orientation (Ellis, 1994). Feminist psychoanalytic supervision includes an understanding of the impact of gender on the client and therapist's construction of self and their relationships with others, including the client–therapist interactions. Similarly, a feminist, reflexive model of discourse analysis encourages the reader to critically examine her subject positionings in relation to the text. However, a discourse analytic reading of text allows a more detailed examina-tion of the complexities involved in the relationship between feminism and psychotherapy as it exposes the ways in which multiple meanings are produced within and by the participants and the framework.

However, understood from a Foucauldian perspective, discourse is not simply a synonym for spoken or written speech, but 'systems of statements which construct an object' (Parker, 1992, p. 5). Discourses both structure meanings and make them available. We are positioned by them and thus acquire subjectivity in relation to them. Consequently, although taking spoken or written text as the focus of analysis enables us to explore variation in accounts or the ways in which positions are constructed, it also reveals the ways in which speakers draw on available discourses to construct meanings or identities. While discourses are multiple, some dominate through their elabo-ration and maintenance by social institutions and their reproduction through social practices in various ways, indicated by the various themes raised by all the chapters in this book. Deconstructing psychotherapy reminds us that, although the task of the therapist is to challenge fixed beliefs or emotions which interfere with clients' psychological wellbeing, 'the metaphor of therapy as healing is an idealization that obscures another metaphor, that therapists manipulate meanings' (Hare-Mustin and Maracek, 1990, p. 48).

So although feminist psychotherapists may disrupt the more obvious gender-specific discourses, in doing this they will be privileging other meanings drawn from feminist theories which are culturally and historically specific. Burman (1992) gives an example of this in her reading of the text of two individual psychotherapy sessions where both therapist and client identify themselves as feminists. She demonstrates how this therapist's attempts to shape a therapeutic discourse occurs within the parameters of a particular feminist framework (Hare-Mustin, 1980). What is interesting is that this configuration involves an attempt to *not* shape – for instance, by avoiding what is seen as the imposition of direct interpretations on to the client. However, the practice of feminist therapy inevitably involves shaping the process as the therapist draws on a discourse which requires her to consider the client's external situation as equally relevant as her internal world. The practitioner's adoption of multiple positions – as 'therapist who knows best' and as 'exploratory feminist' – is highlighted in her fluctuating attempts to enable the client to initiate and explore topics as much as she does, as the therapist. Because discourse analysis refrains from attributing either conscious or unconscious intentions to text, in Burman's reading, we cannot be sure how much the discourse is shaped by the therapeutic orientation of the therapist and how much this is a reflection of her attempt as a feminist to negotiate power and control between herself and her client. Finally, we would also need to reflexively account for the impact of the writer's relationship with the therapist, her position in analysing the session, as well as the positions adopted by readers.

Textual identities

In this section I also use discourse analysis to illustrate some of the practices which function to construct a feminist psychoanalytic model of therapy. However, while elsewhere I have analysed text from my psychotherapy practice (Heenan, 1995b), here I explore an extract from a clinical supervision session in which I am the supervisee. This supervision was self-consciously reflexive in that it also acted as a component of my PhD research project, part of whose focus was to reflexively critique my participation as a group therapist working with women who had eating problems. This involved tape-recording not just the group sessions but the clinical supervision sessions and using discourse analysis to explore text. The extracts are from the third of eight sessions in which I express some of the tensions I experience in promoting a *feminist* perspective within the group. One form this difficulty takes is making me compromise between my theoretical orientation as a psychoanalytic therapist and my political position as a feminist. However, I am equally concerned about the discourse I and my supervisor are generating, referring specifically to the previous session. In a similar vein, Chapter 3 addressed tensions which arise when attempting to work subversively as an educational psychologist.

Although there are many ways in which this text could be approached (Heenan, 1995a), here I am interested in demonstrating how adopting a post-structuralist critique enables us to deepen understanding of the complexities involved in thinking reflexively within a deconstructive framework in order to analyse the gendered dynamics of individual women's distress. In attempting to do this, both the supervisor and the supervisee must adopt multiple positions in relation to each other and the client group. The development of ideas within and between these positions – as feminists, therapists and feminist therapists – illustrates the ways in which therapeutic discourse is produced and reproduced. However, this also challenges and develops theory and practice, highlighting the dynamic and *discursive* nature of the feminist supervisory process which in turn constructs the *feminist* therapeutic process. For in order to shift between particular and, at times, contradictory identities in relation to themselves and the clients, the supervisor and supervisee must move between the very oppositions they are involved in deconstructing; that is, the interior and exterior, the individual and the social, the emotional and intellectual. Attending to the language they employ highlights the dynamic nature of power which they utilize, enact, reject, embody.

1   *Author*: But, it, it's around the whole issue which of course is what my
     project is about which is you know – how do you take a feminist
     approach into the clinic room, in a way, into your actual practice?
     And it – what was sort of bugging me was thinking about um some of
5   the ways we were talking about women – and the way it – I suppose
     the thing that's always driven me crazy in my work which is how, how
     I often, you end up coming to talk about women as sort of, kind of
     slightly immature and kind of um, I, I suppose the whole thing of how
     do you take a kind of perspective that addresses social issues into the
10 individual? And I often, I often used to feel and we used to have
     great arguments – I'm sure this isn't unfamiliar to you at, you know
     at [name of organization] about um, you know how do, just how do
     you do this?
     Supervisor: You mean the interplay between uh, the kind of position
15 that women find themselves in socially and how easily in a kind of
     regular setting that can get pathologized?
     Author: Ya, ya.
     Supervisor: Whereas actually it's, it's clearly about how they've been
     brought up and the culture they've been brought up in.
20 *Author*: Mm, ya.
     Supervisor: And how you can begin to unravel those strands.

From the start, the author constructs a *mutually* problematic discourse for herself and her supervisor as 'psychoanalytic therapists' and 'feminist therapists'. She appeals to the supervisor's identity as 'feminist' therapist (lines 2–3: 'how do you take a feminist approach into the clinic room?'). The shift between her use of 'I' and 'you' in lines 7–8: ('how I often, you end up coming to talk about women as sort of, kind of slightly immature') and her concurrent reference to 'you' in general and 'you' as the other, enables her to ally themselves. The supervisors' response in lines 14–16 ('You mean the interplay between uh, the kind of position that *women* find themselves in socially and how easily in a kind of *regular* setting that can get pathologized?' (author's emphasis)) serves a number of purposes. Clarifying the 'problem' locates it outside the session in that as feminist therapists, they are not 'regular' therapists. Corroborating the author's discourse of feminist therapy as problematic reinforces this by confirming the author's position alongside the supervisor as 'feminist therapist'. While it appears to establish them as colleagues involved together in a problem-solving task, the shift to 'you' in line 21 ('and how you can begin to unravel those strands') could also differentiate the supervisor as 'knowing', from the author who still needs to 'unravel those strands'.

Further, the text illustrates other ambiguities. The supervisor's reference to the gendered identity of the clients as 'women' highlights the existence of this shared feature *between* the two speakers *as well as* with the client group. Nevertheless, questions of inclusion and exclusion in this category then follow: in lines 18–19 ('how *they've* been brought up and the culture *they've* been brought up in' (author's emphasis)). The use of 'they' fails to clarify whether it is a reference to women clients or all women. This also serves to accentuate the different power relations which can be invoked in adopting different social positions: in this instance, the speakers are the 'knowing' therapists and the women are the clients they 'know about'.

While this dialogue creates a distance between the therapists and 'other' women, it also functions to 'begin to unravel those strands' for both the speakers and you, the readers. The difficulties of shifting between the *subject* of themselves as 'feminist therapists' and the *object* of study, 'feminist therapy', indicates some of the tensions which arise in maintaining an actively reflexive stance as both therapist and researcher. While their positions as feminists should enjoin them with (some) other women, their positions as therapists temporarily separate them from clients. The speakers are, at one and the same time, both subject and object, attempting to bridge oppositions between them, yet also constructing them. They continue to 'unravel the strands'.

22 *Author*: Ya, so I often find – and I, you know I don't know if this is familiar to you, that it's very – I find that it's quite easy to talk about it theoretically.
25 *Supervisor*: Mm.
    Author: You know and position women and look at all the, the interplay between these issues.
    Supervisor: Mm, mm.
    Author: I, I find myself sort of slipping into – well, I suppose it's
30 something to do with having an analytic approach, is really slipping into the interior world and never feeling satisfied that I've really kind of brought in these other bits.

Supervisor: It's making some sense but my question is how does that
– how do you think that gets reflected in our discourse?
35 *Author*: Right.
Supervisor: And uh.
Author: Right.
Supervisor: And in your feedback to them – what you're saying to
them?
40 *Author*: Right.
Supervisor: I mean I think it's a really interesting and critical
part.
Author: Well, what I felt that we, we'd got into – and that's why I'm
so annoyed that this thing [referring to the tape recorder which
45 hadn't successfully picked up the last supervision session] didn't
actually work cause I was thinking it would be really helpful to kind
of.
Supervisor: To see the factors in hand.
Author: To have it. But anyway, what I sort of felt that we'd both
50 slipped into, um, is a sort of, is this individualizing of these women
you know – why are they not um – a kind of accusatory way uh, kind
of dialogue.

The supervisor's enquiry: 'How do you think that gets reflected in *our* discourse,' (speaker's emphasis) in line 34, functions to bring the author's attention back to how the speakers may be reproducing the very discourse they are
meant to be transforming. However, by asking the question, it simultaneously
positions the supervisor as someone who need not simply reproduce, but
instead, *could* transform. Although there may be some tensions between
feminism and their model of therapy (lines 29–31: 'Well, I suppose it's something to do with [how] having an analytic approach is really slipping into the
interior world'), the problem is also located *in their dialogue* during the previous session (lines 49–51: 'What I sort of felt that we'd both slipped into, um, is
a sort of, is this individualizing of these women you know'). This extract
illustrates some of the confusing ways in which the term 'discourse' is used
simultaneously: as repertoire, as rhetoric, as social relationship (Burman and
Parker, 1993), demonstrating the fundamental way in which language actively
constructs.

While the speakers clarify their contribution to this reproduction, this text
also illustrates some of the tensions between psychoanalysis and feminism;
'individualizing' reinforces the psychoanalytic framework which focuses on
the interior world of the client. In contrast, feminism clearly emphasizes
deconstructing the difficulties women experience through their status within
the social category of 'woman'. However, it is difficult in this context to keep
the analytic world *out* as is indicated in lines 30–31 ('slipping into the interior
world') and line 50 ('individualizing of these women') and, indeed, the task
here *is* to interweave the inner and the outer. The dialogue also serves to

remind us that 'these women' *are* particular individuals; perhaps they *are* also experiencing unique dilemmas which may not be common to all women? Certainly their positions as members of a psychotherapy group affords them a particular (peculiar?) status. After all, the speakers are therapists whose jobs involve them paying individual attention to their clients in order to enable them to understand and change themselves and their lives. At the same time, as *feminist* therapists, they have a commitment to understanding the interaction between these individual dilemmas and their social situations. So while they separate 'these women therapists' from 'those women clients', like the speakers, 'those clients' also have multiple and changing identities as women and as clients which need to be acknowledged and articulated both by themselves and the therapists. These tensions are also expressed in the double meaning of being a speaking subject – of subjection by language and acquiring subjectivity through language.

The following and final piece of text continues to underline the similarities between the reflexive and interactive framework of feminism, psychoanalysis and the discourse analytic research paradigm.

53 *Supervisor*: But I, I, I. I do remember there being a real sense of frustration.
55 *Author*: Mm, yes.
    Supervisor: Of picking that up.
    Author: Yes.
    Supervisor: From you and this continual thing of you know, how long have we got? Really, are we going to be able to do any good at all for
60 these women and therefore.
    Author: Right, ya.
    Supervisor: That sense of let's hurry it up.
    Author: Yaa.
    Supervisor: So that not only I can see some results in them but you
65 know I have something to put down in my research.
    Author: Ya.
    Supervisor: And I think you mustn't forget that part of it.
    Author: Yes, yes, although, ya, I mean I think that is around although I mean it doesn't matter for the research if the group is a success or
70 not but I'm sure in terms of writing it all down, there's a, there's an element in me that wants it to kind of be successful for that. Um.
    Supervisor: I mean, but also, isn't that exactly what they do to themselves? And probably.
75 *Author*: Ya.
    Supervisor: Don't say, that in fact the more the setting is supposedly feminist, the less they feel able to actually come and voice – I mean I don't know about this particular group but certainly in my experi-

ence at [name of organization]. It's sort of, there are certain things
80   that are like, you can't really mention.
Author: Ya.
Supervisor: It's taboo. I mean of course it isn't but it's very difficult
for them to start saying 'Actually, I just want to go on a diet'.

The supervisor continues to explore the author's complaint. She takes an
actively reflexive stance, first drawing the author's attention to the context of
the therapy group *which is also part of* her research project (lines 64–5: 'so that
not only *I* can see some results in them but you know *I* have something to put
down in my research' (speaker's emphasis)). This reminds the author of their
mutual commitment to a reflexive and discursive approach to therapy as
researchers. Linking the author with the group members (lines 73–4: 'isn't that
exactly what *they* do to themselves?' (speaker's emphasis)), she extends this
reflexive exploration further by inviting the author to consider the impact of
gender on *her* thoughts, feelings and actions in relation to this inclusive
project. This phrase also draws on psychoanalytic intra-psychic concepts which
posit individuals as actively relating to parts of selves, constructing, transforming and constraining aspects of selves.

However, there is a further way in which both speakers are linked with
the group members in that their reflexive exploration of the therapeutic process requires that they focus not just on the clients' unconscious processes but
their own. For although the aim of clinical supervision is not to analyse the
supervisee, a psychoanalytic understanding of the therapeutic relationship
involves the supervisor and supervisee utilizing their conscious and unconscious emotional reactions to clients and, at times, to each other. Thus, while
the supervisor 'stands outside' the therapy, her feelings about the clinical
material being presented and the dynamics of the presentation are often seen
as 'reflectors' of the dynamics of the client–therapist relationship (Heap,
1975). Indeed, some authors describe the dynamics of psychotherapy supervision as a mirror for the therapy being discussed (Langs, 1980). However, it is
clear from this extract that clinical supervision, like language, acts to construct,
not to reflect, thereby 'producing a subject', as Chapter 7 illustrates in relation
to the process of 'statementing' children.

Finally, to come back to an interesting twist in the final piece of text, the
supervisor appears to turn the oppositional tables between feminism and
psychoanalysis. First in lines 76–7, she wonders if, 'in fact the more the setting
is *supposedly* feminist, the less they feel able to actually come and voice'
(author's emphasis)). Then, in lines 82–3, she argues that in a feminist therapy
setting, 'it's very difficult for them [the clients] to start saying, "Actually, I just
want to go on a diet".' These extracts raise a number of questions: is it the
practice of feminist therapy which is oppressive or is it feminism in opposition
to therapy, which is oppressive? What is it that makes it difficult for clients to
'come and voice'? Here we see a shift from the early text where a feminist

perspective was imposed on 'those women' in an overarching way, to an awareness of the way in which *feminist therapy* may be seen as an imposition. Has feminist therapy come to be regulatory in that it does not allow clients to go on reducing diets? Does it measure success in terms of clients subscribing to *its* discursive practices? Does true understanding come from feminist and psychoanalytic theory, not behavioural psychology or health education? Or could it be that the therapist is only 'supposedly' a feminist, thus not offering a truly therapeutic setting – one which is both feminist and therapeutic – in which clients could 'come and voice'?

Deconstructing feminist therapy

Before falling into the solipsistic pit which some critics accuse discourse analysis of digging for itself (Burman and Parker, 1993), I want to locate this specific example of how feminist therapy is constructed within a more general deconstruction of the 'project' of feminist psychotherapy. One of the most serious criticisms of feminist object relations theory is its failure to reflexively locate its adherence to Enlightenment beliefs which presume that it is possible to adopt a position outside the economy, enabling the holder to 'act as the author of one's own subject' (Poovey, 1988). Failing to deconstruct the ways in which they use the overarching category 'woman' (Butler, 1990a) means, for instance, that their views of the mother–daughter relationship privilege Eurocentric norms of 'family', subsuming differences in the ways in which women are reared in matriarchal families and thus how these relationships may be understood, while producing particular notions of femininity (Phoenix, 1987; Spelman, 1988; van Mens-Verhulst, Schreurs and Woertman, 1993).

O'Connor and Ryan (1993) and Chodorow (1994) have further critiqued the way in which psychoanalytic accounts of development uphold and reproduce heterosexuality as the 'norm'. Thus, while feminist therapists would distance themselves from traditional psychotherapists who regard homosexuality or lesbianism as 'something to be cured', they may still not acknowledge or deconstruct erotic feelings between heterosexual women, or between themselves and their female clients, whether heterosexual or lesbian (O'Connor and Ryan, 1993). Flax (1990) is similarly concerned with the way in which the privileging of the mother–daughter relationship in feminist object relations theory shields heterosexuality. However, she extends this critique to show how this also acts to desexualize women and to take attention away from women's sexuality *per se*: heterosexual intercourse which usually precludes birth, erotic feelings between mothers and infants and, in addition, the *bodies* women inhabit.

Despite the proliferation of feminist object relations' writings about women's relationships with their bodies, eating and food, it is the writings of the French Lacanian psychoanalytic feminists, Irigaray, Cixous and Kristeva,[2] which are seen to firmly locate women's subjectivities in bodily experiences; so much so that in particular, Irigaray and Cixous have been accused of falling prey to essentialist beliefs which work to reduce women to nothing but bodies (Weedon, 1987). In spite of this, Weedon (1987, p. 70) describes the appeal of Kristeva's perspective:

> it is Kristeva's theory of the subject as unstable, in process and constituted in language which is of most interest to a feminist post-structuralism. This radical alternative to the humanist view of subjectivity, in which it is self-present, unified and in control, offers the possibility of understanding the contradictory nature of individuals and of their dispersal across a range of subject positions of which they are not the authors.

Spelman (1988) adds another dimension to critiques of object relations theory. She argues that it is *not* able to fully account for the social conditions in which individual gendered subjectivity is constructed; its microcosmic focus on the mother–infant dyad does not locate this relationship in terms of their multiple social positions as 'raced' and 'classed', thus rendering it an *asocial* theory of gender relations. By posing a false separation between gender, race and class or other social inequalities, it functions to privilege gender oppression above and beyond other social inequalities, a criticism which McLeod (1994) also makes of the practice of feminist therapy. Moreover, it means that irrespective of which woman is 'other' to the norm presumed by feminist therapists, she is critiqued from a perspective which functions to maintain difference as 'otherness' to an assumed 'normality'.

So the answer to one of the questions raised in the previous text: 'Isn't that exactly what *they* do to themselves?' (lines 73–4) depends on which discourse of subjectivity the therapist employs at any particular moment. Those employed by feminist object relations psychotherapists are subsumed within a prevailing contemporary Western discourse which positions the client as agentic and intentional, from birth to adulthood (Mahoney and Yngvesson, 1992). This highlights another tension within the project of feminist therapy which has not yet been made explicit by reference to the text; this is the problematic way in which therapy positions the client as 'responsible'. While a client clearly is *not* responsible for the circumstances of her birth or her family's social or cultural position, by virtue of entering psychotherapy and exploring conscious and unconscious processes, the client enters into a world in which she then *becomes* responsible for taking the steps necessary to change her adult relationships with others or parts of herself.

In spite of these tensions, some feminist post-structuralists see psychoanalytic concepts as opening up possible ways of understanding subjectivities. For instance, Elshtain (1982) argues that drawing on notions of the unconscious, or defence mechanisms such as splitting, projection or displacement, could contribute towards developing a more complex and thus thorough model of the mind than the dualistic notions which have come out of Enlightenment theories. This would be 'an account that unites mind and body, reason and passion, into a compelling account of human subjectivity and identity, and the creation of a feminist theory of action that, complicatedly, invokes both inner and outer realities' (p. 618). Flax (1990) further suggests that the appeal of Enlightenment beliefs in the superiority of mind over body could be better understood by utilizing psychoanalytic concepts such as the primitive defence mechanism of 'splitting'. The appeal of privileging singular perspectives, even privileging post-structuralist beliefs, could also be recognized as an illustration of an infantile omnipotent desire 'to know'; that is, to 'have *one* truth' versus multiple realities.

The practice of reflexively reading text from a feminist clinical supervision marks a shift from abstract theoretical analysis, so typical of discussions of deconstruction. By focusing on the dynamic and discursive ways in which theoretical concepts are deployed in practice, it makes visible the way in which multiple meanings are produced and reproduced by the feminist therapists' theoretical and political framework. In turn, this mirrors the shifting, contradictory way in which selves are presented in psychotherapy. At the same time, the speakers are very 'real' selves, involved in an ongoing critique and negotiation of their positions and practices, just as their clients' selves are also real, in contrast to the feminist heroines (Bordo, 1988) or the passive victims (McLeod, 1994) which feminist object relations theory is accused of constructing.

Indeed, you the reader will also have a mixture of ways of approaching and understanding this dialogue, just as you will have varied ways of interacting with my analysis. Needless to say, as author I operate from a privileged position in terms of selecting text and ascribing meaning. This is explicitly marked in the shifts of self-reference between 'I', 'she', 'her', 'the author', 'the speaker' or 'the supervisee'. However, as 'the therapist', my reading of the text includes an assumption of the existence and operation of unconscious processes. So, for instance, in the final piece of text when I say, 'I'm sure in terms of writing it all down, there's a, there's an element in me that wants it to kind of be successful for that' (lines 70–1), I am referring to my feelings about this very public process of writing for an audience.

This attention to deconstruction is one link between feminist psychoanalytic theory and post-structuralist accounts. However, a post-structuralist critique of feminist therapy's 'claims to knowledge' acts to further deconstruct not only the object of its knowledge – woman – but also the epistemological underpinnings of its theory and practice. At the same time, some feminist post-structuralists draw on psychoanalytic notions such as unconscious processes and defence mechanisms, in order to develop more complex understandings of the construction of subjectivities and the endurance of philosophical positions. Both post-structuralist and therapeutic theories focus on the constructive centrality of language. Adopting a reflexive discourse analysis is one tool which enables us to explore the tensions inherent within the practice of feminist therapy.

Feminist object relations theory offers post-structuralists a model for understanding the complex way in which internal panopticons operate (Bartky, 1988). In particular, their accounts of the impact of gender on women's relationships with psychosocial development demonstrates how women have been made 'fragmented other' to 'rational man' by virtue of being subjected to multiple, shifting disjointed images of themselves – of particular women. However, they have kept their focus on the effects of gender, not acknowledging the way in which either psychotherapeutic or feminist theories act simultaneously as liberators and regulators. Although feminist object relations theory has sustained a great deal of criticism in terms of its failure to deconstruct its own subject, these writers' commitment to deconstructing gendered aspects of *psychoanalytic* theory and practice may offer a more enduring means to further understand 'woman' than their counterparts, the feminist 'empowerment' psychotherapists. The wholesale way in which texts like Worell and Remer's (1992) proudly describe how feminist 'empowerment' therapies have been taken on board by the psychological professions in North America suggests that, rather than representing a challenge to the practice of mainstream psychology, they are instead being subsumed by them as another way in which to market their product as truly applicable to all. Chapter 5 highlights how the National Health Service in Britain attempts to market its services to black women.

Rather than *applauding* the existence of an organization like the 'Advanced Feminist Therapy Institute' (cited from Dutton-Douglas and Walker, 1988), I worry about it. Doubtless, this is partly out of envy because it has only taken this group of women *five* years to label themselves as 'advanced' feminist therapists, whereas I am still struggling to understand how to put this concept into practice after more than 12 years. On a more serious level, my worry is more to do with the way in which an overarching notion of feminism has been applied to the practice of therapies which have been rendered 'good for women' by virtue of having been deemed suitable for *the* feminist cause. This institutionalization of feminist therapy serves to remind us not just how some forms of feminism have become woven into consumerism, but also of the pervasiveness of discourse: feminism in this singular form is *also* a discourse.

Notes

1 For a more complete discussion of feminist object relations theory, see Chodorow, 1989.
2 See Grosz, 1989, for a fuller account of Kristeva and Irigaray.

Part II

Practising (at) the limits of representation

The next three chapters set out to challenge categories and constructions which are characteristically (re)produced within research and practice settings. In particular, they challenge the ways such categories homogenize, essentialize and naturalize as individual, psychological qualities what are features of people's historical and current circumstances. Whether in relation to women (patients in high security mental hospitals, Chapter 6), black women (in mental health services) (Chapter 5), or young people's exclusions from mainstream schools (Chapter 7), the process of categorization is shown to limit and prescribe the available identities and activities; of ourselves as practitioners, as well as of those to whom we aim to be (or are institutionally positioned as being) of service. As practitioners, we often find ourselves positioned as working with clients in two extreme contexts: of either pathological representation/overrepresentation or with total absence of representation.

Constructs of 'gender' (Chapters 5 and 6), 'race' (Chapter 5) and 'school exclusion' (Chapter 7) have been defined by the dominant/powerful knowledge-producing agencies and are generally treated as coherent and uncontestable. In this part we show how such definitions become reified and naturalized as 'facts'. This process achieves three effects. First, it conceals their status as social productions; second, it obscures the prescriptions made by such legitimized power relations; and, third, it inevitably shapes social practices which in turn require the reproduction or reconstruction of those very categories to maintain the status quo. Indeed, categories of mad/abused women, black women and 'school disruptors' are both visible in their absence (as in the under-representation of black women in mental health services, Chapter 5), but are also confined, constrained and/or pathologized where they are present (as women in special hospitals, Chapter 6; young adults excluded from school, Chapter 7).

Key questions about who benefits from such processes of representation are themselves in danger of being transformed and confined within an equivalently reified opposition of good and bad. Yet as Chapters 6 and 7 illuminate, the instability of such definitions can easily be seen in people's accounts of their lived experiences, as well as by attending to fluctuations in the careers of particular categories employed by dominant groups at particular historical timepoints. Thus the chapters in this section underscore how people do not easily fit into simplistic representations of the available constructed categories: women are not simply adjuncts to men (Chapter 6), women, including black women, are not an homogeneous, gendered or racialized group (Chapter 5), the child subjects of 'school exclusions' are variably positioned as passive or active, as responsible or victimized, or as rebellious, remorseful or grateful (Chapter 7). Thus all the chapters attempt to illuminate the shifting and multiple potential of attending to these different (albeit constructed) positions.

The title of this section of the book, 'Practising (at) the limits of representation', highlights how practitioner-experts of 'the psy complex' both work inside existing conceptual frameworks and also by their practice help to define and maintain those categories' entry into representation. Practices of representation structure how experiences are understood; they define and constrain the range of possible positions. We see professional practices (here of clinical, educational and academic psychology) as policing the boundaries of dominant social categories (such as those of gender, 'race', age, sexuality – and above all of normality) and as such they contribute to the structures of visibility and exclusion they perpetuate. Those of us who live and/or make our living at these borders of what is (allowed to be) known need to work together, not only to reinterpret what our practices (dis)allow but also to change what it is we/they do.

Chapter 5

The present absence/pathologized presence of black women in mental health services

Gill Aitken

Introduction

The National Health Service (NHS) has been in a state of flux and transition since 1989 when the government set out to alter drastically the basis of Britain's healthcare provision (*Health Journal*, 1989). This chapter is particularly concerned with the government's focus on black mental health issues, whereby statutory (mental) health service purchasers and providers have been challenged to move away from a service model which provides for an assumed homogeneous (white) population to one which meets the needs of multicultural contemporary British society (Department of Health, 1993a). The establishment of both the Ethnic Health Unit (EHU) and the Regional 'Race' Programme (RRP) in 1994 could be seen to signal the government's active commitment to 'race' issues within the NHS. For example, throughout its proposed three-year lifespan, one specific aim of the EHU is to secure greater benefit for black and 'ethnic' minority people in England from the NHS (Chan, 1995), whilst the RRP's remit is to develop national consultative procedures and programmes with representatives of black and/or 'ethnic' minority groups (NHS Task Force, 1994a, 1994b).

Such recommendations and initiatives have been generally welcomed, despite a number of reservations. For example, previous attempts to redress racial inequities in Britain (e.g. the Race Relations Act 1976) have not significantly changed the Eurocentric bias of policies and practices and the material circumstances of black peoples relative to white remains largely unchanged (e.g. Bhat, Carr-Hill and Ohri; 1988; Torkington, 1991; Ahmad, 1992; Wheeler, 1994). Moreover, there is an additional problem of theorizing the relationships between different forms of oppressions/inequalities. Within the 'race' debate, 'gender' issues appear to be largely subordinated to those relating to 'race', 'ethnicity' and 'culture'.[1] The question therefore arises as to the particular implications for black women's position in relation to mental health.

The underlying assumption of the government seems to be that there will be collaboration and shared understanding of, and commitment to, such changes by individuals, professions and institutions alike. Largely absent is any explicit critical discussion and understanding of the wider socio-historico-political contexts within which black peoples – and black women in particular – are positioned and the implications for future statutory mental health service provision. These form the topic of this chapter, which is divided into two main sections. In the first, I review how black women and men and white women have been historically (mis)represented through the construction and regulation of discourses on 'race' and 'gender'. Using illustrative examples, I explore how the production of essentialized concepts of 'race' and 'gender' characteristically construct such social groups as the undifferentiated 'other'. Yet under particular socio-historico-political conditions this has been used to differentiate among and between women and 'races', and this continues to the present day. In the second section, I review black women's present statistical representation and visibility both as providers and users of statutory mental health services. Both their presence and invisibility relative to other socially constructed groups will be illuminated by relating this to the dominant discursive 'homogeneous' representations of black peoples, white women and Black women themselves (see also Anthias and Yuval-Davis, 1993). I argue that the British government's reliance on increased statistical representation of 'ethnic' groups to redress pre-existing inequalities has limitations in particular for black women's positions.

It should be noted that the proposed government changes are to take place within an NHS which is an increasingly complex organization comprising multiple administrative levels and clinical specialisms and professions. Underpinned by the (assumed) medico-scientific basis of its discipline (Littlewood, 1991), psychiatry has established itself as being ultimately responsible for the clinical assessment, diagnosis and medicalized management of 'mental illness' either independently of, or increasingly (and sometimes uneasily) coexisting with, other emergent disciplines of (clinical) psychology, psychotherapy and counselling. While these latter disciplines may focus on the psychological assessment and management of mental illness, in common with psychiatry they continue to establish their scientific credentials in articulating their rights to manage mental illness by stressing the objective and/or scientific underpinning of theories, research and practice (Fernando, 1991; Alladin, 1992; Good, 1994), rather than challenging their ideological bases (see also this volume, Chapters 3 and 7).

The objective and scientific bases of such disciplines and professions have been increasingly contested over the last 30 years by a number of anti-racist and feminist practitioners, researchers and user groups. They have argued that these disciplines function to reflect, shape and justify particular economic, political and social orders and ideologies (see e.g. Black Health Workers and Patients Group, 1983; Caplan and Gans, 1991; Ussher, 1991; Ahmad, 1993) and operate as specific methods of control and punishment of black women (and black men) in particular (Sayal, 1990; Torkington, 1991; Fernando, 1993a, 1993b).

Thus an alternative and growing literature debates and illuminates the androcentric and Eurocentric biases of psychiatry and psychology and associated research and practices (Fernando, 1991; Torkington, 1991; Webb-Johnson, 1991; Bhavnani and Phoenix, 1994; Mama, 1995). Black feminists, in particular, have noted the non-gendered perspective of much of the anti-racist literature and argued that the focus on 'gender' has been largely based on white middle-class women's concerns (Marshall, 1994; Wheeler, 1994; Mama, 1995). As Collins (1990) more generally highlights: 'white feminists identify with their [black women's] victimisation as women yet ignore the privilege that racism grants them . . . Black men decry racism yet see sexism as being less objectionable.' Historically whether referring to mainstream mental health, anti-racist or white feminist bodies of knowledge, black women have been largely edited out, subsumed within the concerns of black men or white feminists, and/or excluded from involvement in the setting of agendas for policies, research and practices. Consequently, there has been little systematic research undertaken with black women and for black women in relation to mental health (Sayal, 1990).

However, when black women are constituted as a category, they are generally defined by others and 'looked at from the outside' (Fernando, 1993a, p. 53), being seen as constitutive of specific homogeneous and polarized 'race' and 'gender' categories (Afshar and Maynard, 1994). Yet it has been shown that black women may expect particular subordinations shaped by class and 'gender' specificities (see for example, Wheeler, 1994; Mama, 1995). Black women's positioning as subordinate not only to white men, but also under particular circumstances and at particular times to white women and black men has effectively ensured that in contemporary Britain they remain a minority within a minority (see e.g. Wheeler, 1994), with racism and sexism interrelating to produce 'race'-specific gender effects (Dugger, 1991). Some authors have argued that black women, who are likely to experience multiple discrimination and disadvantage, are least likely to have their needs met in relation to mental health issues (Williams and Watson, 1993).

As a white woman, during my present training and practice within the predominantly white profession of clinical psychology within the NHS (1993–1996), it has become clear to me that the historically and socially constructed opposition between whiteness and blackness, and between male and female, has produced systems of domination which are reproduced within the training for and practices of statutory mental health service professions. Black women are effectively rendered 'officially' invisible as both providers and users of, for example, clinical psychology services. Moreover, the privileges and assumptions which arise from my own 'whiteness' and the 'whiteness' of my discipline and profession have not been a focus of my training (Wong, 1994). Such experiences are arguably not specific to clinical psychology but are general to education, training and employment within Britain (e.g. Brah, 1991; Torkington, 1991; (charles), 1992; Wong, 1994).

I am not arguing that the existence and perpetuation of racist and sexist ideologies is specific to mental health professions, such as psychiatry and clinical psychology (Fernando, 1993a, 1993b). However, if as practitioners and/or researchers in this field we ignore how existing concepts, assumptions and theories associated with 'race' and 'gender' have been (re)produced, legitimated, disseminated, applied and experienced and fail to raise the fundamental question of 'who benefits from these?', then the degree to which 'significant' changes as proposed by the government can be effected may be limited. Throughout the following sections, using illustrative examples, I review how under the changing conditions of colonialism, patriarchy and capitalism the shifting and connecting constructions of 'race' and 'gender' have operated to maintain pre-existing systems of dominant–subordinate relations. From the eighteenth century these have increasingly depended on scientific and individualistic discourses (and the use of classificatory practices) for their legitimation and dissemination. Such constructions continue to be used to exclude, marginalize and/or problematize black women within 'wider' British society; and these are (re)produced within NHS structures in general and in psychiatry and (clinical) psychology in particular. At a time when the NHS is becoming a competitive market place, with professions and disciplines attempting to establish and protect credentials and the rights to manage different aspects of healthcare, of which of 'mental illness' is one aspect, it may be that the appropriation and refinement of oppressive ideologies and practices, rather than the identification and challenging of oppressive assumptions, practices and structures may predominate.

Before proceding further, I should clarify two issues. First, I use the term 'black' as a political category and as a marker of the exploitation by white British peoples through European slavery practices from the fifteenth century (e.g. Yeboah, 1988). The term embraces all peoples with origins from within the African, Indian and West Indian continents, but is not intended to obscure the diversity, multiplicity or dynamic aspects of black peoples' own self-identifications or experiences. Moreover, alongside the specificities of the socially constructed relations associated with the terms 'race' and 'gender', 'class' issues also figure in intersecting and non-reducible ways (e.g. Brah, 1992).

Second, I focus on the ways in which representations of specific social categories have been produced in the attempt to continually privilege certain sectors of (white) British society. Thus regulation and control by dominant groups in white British society appears as a key theme throughout. However, black peoples and women in general, and black women in particular, share histories of developing a range of strategies of resistance in surviving and challenging multiple oppressions. Throughout I attempt to refer readers to literatures which make such strategies more clearly visible.

The construction of essentialized 'racialized' and 'genderized' differences

Over the centuries, the concept and construction of 'differences' between and among peoples, and the composition and status of such groups, has been subject to the changing and competing influences of various privileged institutions (e.g. monarchy, church, science) and discourses (e.g. superstitious, religious, scientific, moral, political, and economic). In Britain, as a number of complex social, economic and political phenomena arose out of the changing conditions of slavery, colonialism, capitalism and patriarchy, various accounts have documented how particularly from the seventeenth century there was an increasing shift from a reliance on religious discourses to 'scientific' discourses and institutions to reinforce, reproduce and legitimate the genderization and racialization of social practices within society (e.g. Rose, Lewontin and Kamin, 1984; Yeboah, 1988; Littlewood and Lipsedge, 1989; Ussher, 1991; Ahmad, 1993; Fernando, 1993a; Mama, 1995). Of particular relevance to the present chapter is how the concepts of 'rationality' and 'reason' (on which science is predicated) came to be situated within the 'individual' and constructed as a fundamental signifier of humanity, social order and civilization. Moreover, the possession of rationality became inherently imbued with credibility and legitimacy not only for the production of knowledge, but also with the authority to govern the irrational 'other/s' (Donovan, 1991; Oliver, 1991).

The criteria for possession of 'rationality' has come to be largely based on the 'ability' to be categorized as a white, middle/upper-class male and on the activities of masculinity (Arditti, 1982; Oliver, 1991; Tavris, 1993). As a number of authors have identified, the essentialization of 'differences', and the proclaimed objective and scientific methods of classification and observation has proved vital in the process of reinforcing, reproducing and legitimizing hierarchies which positioned white (middle/upper) class men at the apex of social, economic and political orders. However, such methods have been shown to largely obscure and mystify the self-serving economic, political and social interests of those benefiting from the practices of slavery, capitalism, colonialism and patriarchy (Yeboah, 1988; Essed, 1991; Tavris, 1993; Ahmad, 1993; Mama, 1995).

Following West and Zimmerman's (1991) argument on gender, the ascription of peoples to particular social categories can be seen to prescribe the 'biological inevitability' of gendered (e.g. motherhood) and racialized (e.g. slave/servant) activities. Moreover, genderized and/or racialized activities have been further constructed as the prototypical expression of such category membership. Categorization and activity thus reinforce each other's essentialization, as well as the essentialization of differences between males and females (West and Zimmerman, 1991) and black and white. In being identified as 'different from' (characteristically based on constructed anatomical differences) and perhaps most importantly the evaluative 'lesser than' white male, black women and men (and white women) have been consistently positioned as inherently 'other' – emotional, lesser/non-human, closer to nature.

Representations of blackness and femaleness over the centuries have reflected physical, sexual, mental or moral danger (Oliver, 1991; Marshall, 1994) and have been posed as a threat both to those of us so categorized as well as to the rest of humanity (see e.g. Gilman, 1992, for an account of the construction of black and white female sexuality in the nineteenth century). As women of whichever 'race', throughout history we can find ourselves multiply constructed within the various (shifting and changing) dichotomous categories originally imposed on us: madonna–whore; childlike–motherlike; dependent–emasculating/superwoman; emotional–castrating/non-rational; frigid–animalistic/erotic; passive–aggressive; feminine–unfeminine. Under certain conditions such categories may have been used to exoticize us, but they always pathologize and objectify us. Moreover, women located within particular 'race' and class positions have consistently found themselves placed at ends of the dichotomies and further pathologized/differentiated from other categories of women. For example, under particular circumstances any woman can find herself positioned as whore; the source of disease/corruption. Under other conditions relative to white, middle-class women, white working-class women may find themselves positioned more consistently as whore. Black women, however, are more likely to be constructed as super-whore as well as the prototypical female who is the source of all disease and/or corruption (Ussher, 1991; Gilman, 1992; Marshall, 1994). It is notable that such representations and their incorporation in racist and sexist ideologies both in the past and in the present become particularly visible in public and political arenas. They are used as justification for the 'natural' positions of women and black peoples in society when the assumptions, structures and practices underpinning white male power and practices have been challenged (as in the anti-slavery movements of the eighteenth–nineteenth centuries; the universal suffrage movements of the nineteenth–twentieth centuries; and civil rights movements of the twentieth century). Such representations and discourses arguably target black peoples and white women in the identification, explanation and/or justification of the forms of regulation/ punishment if the stability of society is perceived as threatened, or for the otherwise 'inexplicable' or 'unreasonable' social and personal crises identified by primarily white males. However, at other times, irrespective of 'race' and 'class', any woman may draw on such representations and discourses to legitimate personal and specific social groups' interests which, as Cohen (1988) argues, protect us from recognizing the conditions of our own subordination.

The competing, coexisting and sometimes contradictory discourses of femininity which emerged under the changing conditions of capitalism, slavery, colonialism and patriarchy have acted to legitimize specific and limited forms of institutions (e.g. marriage, motherhood, family), roles (e.g. moral and emotional guardians of society, family) and societal relations (subordinating the needs of women to those of men and children). They have been identified by various feminists in the universal oppression of women irrespective of class and 'race' (Daly, 1979). However, black feminists such as Collins (1990) have questioned the universality of such claims and the relevance of white feminists analyses to black women's experiences. For example, the practices of slavery robbed African women of the rights to their bodies, children, husbands/partners and lands in inhumane ways that white, middle-class women would be unlikely to experience. Moreover, the coexisting actual or symbolic 'demasculinization' of black men ranging from castration to inadequate economic payment for their labour and unemployment has since the times of slavery effectively ensured that many black women have never experienced the same choice as white, middle-class women of being able to rely on males to economically provide for a family. Relatedly, the strategies for survival and resistance of black women who may head lone-parent households have in turn been used to construct the women as contributing to the symbolic demasculinization of black men (Wallace, 1990; Mama, 1995). While white, middle-class women (who were positioned as the ideal guardians of and breeders for society; Bland, 1982) campaigned for the rights of women to birth control and abortion, other categories of women found and continue to find themselves constructed as contributing to the degeneration of humanity (Gilman, 1992). Whether under the conditions of slavery in the fifteenth century or the conditions of a welfare state in the twentieth century, black women and (other) economically disadvantaged women share a history of resisting the enforced removal of and separation from their children as well as enforced birth control and abortion as mediated by representatives (including slave-traders, social workers, health workers, police, judiciary, immigration officers) of the dominant white groups in society.

Thus under particular historical circumstances associated with the conditions of capitalism and colonialism, (conforming) white, middle-class women have found themselves placed higher in the social hierarchy relative to black women or men and/or working-class women. During the period of imperialist expansion, identified 'civilized' white women and 'civilized' practices were held up as exemplars, to be emulated and admired, and which positioned white women in their own 'civilizing' missions in the colonies – whether as imperialists and/or feminists (Chaudhuri and Strobel, 1992; Ware, 1992; Liddle and Rai, 1993).

Examples abound of attempts to divide black peoples to the advantage of dominant white groups' interests. The white British attempted to form 'paternalistic' alliances with a minority of black peoples in the colonies who could assist Britain in administering indirect and direct colonial rule (Chaudhuri and Strobel, 1992). Although the acceptance and internalization of white norms could enable differentiation from the 'mass uncivilized other', the inherent legitimate privileged status and practices of the colonizers remained largely unchallenged. More recently, as Britain has witnessed diverse patterns of migration of peoples from British (former) colonies from 1945, black peoples in Britain have found themselves constructed on the one hand as an homogeneous 'immigrant' group and the cause of the social, economic and welfare deprivation experienced by the 'assumed indigenous British' white populations (Cohen, 1988). On the other hand they may find themselves ascribed to one of two discrete but assumed homogeneous categories of African–Caribbean or Asian (both still problematized in relation to white Britons) and set against each other in terms of their ability to integrate and contribute to British society. Thus people of Afro–Caribbean origins have historically found themselves constructed as too aggressive and of a violent/criminal disposition whereas people of Asian origins have characteristically found themselves constructed as law-abiding, but passive and not prepared to fully integrate into white British society (Carr-Hill and Drew, 1988; Cohen, 1988; Parmar, 1988; Webb-Johnson, 1991) – though this may be changing with the 'Asian riot' (or uprising!) which occured in Bradford in 1995.

It has been argued that the effect of such representations and discourses over the centuries has been to maintain and legitimitize layers of segregation within British society, which continues in contemporary Britain, whereby the rational is positioned to control the irrational (Oliver, 1991). Some authors argue that the white male public world (paid high status employment/higher education system/science) can be differentiated from the white female private (domestic and emotional caring) worlds, with the subordinated servicing of both these worlds by black peoples. Black peoples have typically been marginalized to yet another world: socially, economically, politically and psychologically distanced by the white world, but wherein gendered relations are re-enacted, having particular consequences for black women (Wheeler, 1994; Chatterjee, 1995).

The role of psychiatry and psychology

Since their emergence in the eighteenth century, psychiatry and associated mental health disciplines have coexisted with wider social attempts to refine racist and sexist ideologies in an attempt to justify existing political and economic dominance and unequal power structures (Fernando, 1991; Yeboah, 1988). It has been argued that the institution of psychiatry (and associated professions) has appropriated and constructed discourses and practices which could be largely incorporated within existing valued ideologies. By imposing rationality and scientific order on to a new homogeneous group of the 'mentally ill', psychiatry and psychology could draw on and reconstitute existing knowledge and reframe this 'new' knowledge as scientific/medical/objective thus ensuring its credibility and legitimacy while dismissing alternative knowledges as non-scientific/irrational (Miller and Rose, 1986).

The power of psychiatrists to diagnose 'madness' and to construct a new social group has been seen to signal another form of physical, economic and political segregation between the rational (self) and the irrational (other) (Scull, 1979). The continual refinement of racialized and gendered discourses arguably act as preconditions to position women and black peoples as particularly vulnerable to be diagnosed as 'mad' – but typically within sub-classifications of mental illness which support dominant ideologies (Ussher, 1991; Fernando, 1993b; Sashidharan and Francis, 1993).

Since their emergence, psychiatry and psychology have closely allied themselves to other 'scientific' subdisciplines of biology, somatology, phreno-logy, anatomy, medicine and genetics to establish their biosocial scientific credibility. They can be seen to have actively contributed to the attempts to legitimize the inherent inferiority of both black peoples and white women. A review of the 'scientific' literature, which particularly treats 'race' or 'sex'/ 'gender' as 'independent variables' reveals that theories of biological and cultural transmission proliferate in the search to prove the essential 'differ-ence/s' between black and white peoples, men and women. No aspect of black peoples (and few aspects of the white woman's) body or behaviour appears to have been left untouched in this quest. For example, hair, brain, skulls, limbs, facial features, posteriors, women's labia, men's penises have all been meas-ured, weighed, mutilated in people's lifetimes or on death; reaction times and responses to pain have been recorded in the search to identify differences in the name of 'science'.

The identification and quantification of 'differences' has increasingly re-lied on the employment and refinement of standardized methods of 'scientific' classification, measurement and statistical analyses, particularly since the nine-teenth century. The production of statistically significant differences has proved vital in further scientizing research findings (that studies which do not produce such differences tend not to be published, or many journals are 'controlled' by white, middle-class scientists is largely overlooked – see e.g. Rose, Lewontin and Kamin, 1984) The development and (ab)use of standard-ized IQ tests which rely heavily on Western concepts of intelligence and statistical methods have perhaps been the subject of most controversial public and professional debate in relation to 'race', gender and class issues since their introduction in the early twentieth century. The consistent production and publication of studies which report allegedly significantly higher IQ scores (and/or different score profiles) of white (middle-class) peoples relative to 'others' have often been associated with, or appropriated by, movements and institutions who have sought legitimation of particular social practices which attempt to effectively control 'unfit' peoples' reproductive and productive labour, as well as the distribution of economic and social resources within Britain (Rose, Lewontin and Kamin, 1984; Yeboah, 1988).

The continuity of the construction of black peoples as 'inferior' is still very much in evidence in the 1990s, not only in popular discourses but also mediated by professional journals and texts. As an illustrative example,

I report on work published by Rushton and printed in the *The Psychologist*, the monthly journal of the professional representative body of British psychologists (the British Psychological Society) which is distributed to all its members.

In the process of deciding the extent to which I should refer to Rushton's work, I am aware that I could be publicizing the very myths of which I am so critical and contributing to his citation index (which contributes to a researcher's professional status). However, in this context of critiquing his work (which will not be entered in the reference list),[2] I trust this account will rather facilitate readers to identify and resist the production, articulation and/or publication of such representations and constructions of black peoples (and 'others') in future personal, social or professional lives.

In Table 5.1 below, rather than incorporate some of the absolute figures which Rushton reported, I have modified his data to produce relative rank orderings of a sample of the (non-gendered) data he produced for the three alleged 'races' of 'mongoloids', 'caucasians' and 'negroids'. He proposes that the presented data proves how the supposedly genetic based r(fecundity)/K(parental care) (his terms) evolutionary theory comes closest

Table 5.1: The relative positions of three 'races' in relation to their alleged possession of alleged objective measures of various characteristics.

	'MONGOLOIDS'		'CAUCASIANS'	'NEGROIDS'	
Brain Weight & Intelligence					
Cranial capacity	Greatest	1	2	3	Lowest
IQ	Highest	1	2	3	Lowest
Personality & Temperament					
Aggression	Lowest	3	2	1	Highest
Dominance	Lowest	3	2	1	Highest
Maturation Rate					
Gestation time	Longest	N/A	2	1	Shortest
Reproductive Effort					
Androgen levels	Lowest	3	2	1	Highest
Permissive attitudes	Least	3	2	1	Greatest
Sexually transmitted diseases	Lowest	3	2	1	Highest
Intercourse frequency	Lowest	3	2	1	Highest
Size of genitalia	Smallest	3	2	1	Largest
Social Organization					
Marital stability	Highest	1	2	3	Lowest
Mental health	Highest	1	2	3	Lowest
Law abidingness	Highest	1	2	3	Lowest

(adapted from Rushton, 1990)

to explaining 'race' differences. That he reports that this theory has also been successfully applied in studies of animal and plant differences is presumably intended to further emphasize the objectivity of the presented work. Flynn in the same journal 'rationally' critiques Rushton's work on scientific grounds. He is concerned that the abuse Rushton has received is in danger of preventing this work from getting a hearing in the future. Flynn claims that this is wrong in itself, as 'telling the truth as you see it can never be racist' and may also silence those who believe they can make a reasoned case against Rushton (Flynn, 1989, p. 363, but see also Zuckerman and Brody, 1988, for an alternative – better – form of 'scientific critique'). Such a claim, however, ignores the debates about what constitutes 'truth', and that black peoples' perspectives are largely absent in white-dominated scientific journals.

Although Rushton presents his work as scientific, objective and politically neutral, from Table 5.1 readers can see that the terminology employed (as in the construction of 'races'), the use of 'superordinate constructs' such as stable social organization and the operationalization of these through specific measures such as 'marital stability' ignores the social, political and economic contexts within which the 'researcher' and the 'researched' find themselves. The category of 'race' is reified, designating peoples into three broad and assumed homogeneous categories. In such ways the representations and constructions of black peoples now dating back centuries are reiterated, with white peoples accorded, through alleged scientific evidence, inherent anatomical, biological, psychological and social superiority. It should be noted that such claims cannot now be made without associations of eugenics (genocidal 'final solutions' and notions of 'ethnic cleansing') and Fascism.

If we imagine the bell-shaped 'normal' distribution curve so beloved of statisticians, with white peoples' consistent position of occupying the middle position, whites are constructed as normal, whereas the 'others' possess excess or deficits in characteristics.[3] For example, should the data for 'whites' and 'orientals' (Flynn's, 1989 term) be compared, then it will not be that the latter possess more of the valued characteristics, rather they possess excess. Indeed, 'orientals' are typically devalued for inherently possessing a lack of individuality, which is so valued in Western society. The classification system is so constructed that whichever way we look at it, it confirms white superiority. Theories of intergenerational genetic or cultural transmission of characteristics 'naturally' provide the backdrop for the inevitability of the continuance of such characteristics.

Such studies bolster the factual status of such social (and contestable) constructs of family instability, mental illness and criminality. They treat these as reducible to either biology or culture, which are by inference inherited and inherently associated with black peoples. It is no mere coincidence that these same phenomena are ones which have been identified by, at least, the present British government as contemporary social problems and a burden on economic resources, as it engages in the process of dismantling our 'welfare state', while at the same time promoting individual responsibility and account-ability (see also Chapter 3).

So, for example, the selection and inclusion of measures such as inter-course frequency, gestation times and numbers of children feed into discourses of sexuality which since the times of slavery have positioned black men as both sexual 'studs' and rapists, black women as promiscuous, corruptors and/or breeders and both black women and men as 'animal like'. Overall, black people have been portrayed as a continuing threat to the existence of the 'civilized' white 'race' and over the centuries this threat has been variously articulated as: degeneracy (e.g. if transracial offspring are produced); as white people being numerically overwhelmed if numbers of black peoples remain unchecked; and as the transmission of disease and destruction – from the social hygiene movements of the nineteenth century to AIDS in the late twentieth century. In turn, such discourses can be seen to legitimize systems of regula-tion and have implications for the forms of social control to be used – particu-larly focusing on physical or coercive forms of regulation as in the (mental) health and judicial systems. These include sterilization, birth control, the use of major tranquillizers and sectioning[4] under the Mental Health Acts. Evi-dence of 'mental illness' has also been specifically linked to immigration controls with proposals for repatriation (Rack, 1982). Finally, the association of 'intelligence' with other characteristics, including the construct of 'race', also functions to legitimize the definition of acceptable roles for black peoples, in that they are assumed as not being capable of societally valued intellectual activity and are thus excluded from the production of knowlege/power and denied legitimate authority to challenge existing dominant forms of knowledge.

Although some may argue that Rushton's account is an extreme case example (but recall its automatic circulation to all members of the British Psychological Society), the search for and confirmation of essentialized differences between black and white peoples is still evident in the majority of mainstream psychology and psychiatric journals and texts, whether promoted as grounded in either biological or cultural differences. Further, as 'scientists' attempt to incorporate the discourses of egalitarianism, it may be that when 'race' issues are referred to, more subtle forms of racism may occur which require 'a degree of sensitivity rather than awareness alone to decipher and articulate it' (Owusu-Bempah and Howitt, 1994, p. 166).

Based on the above overview of the constructions of 'race' and gender, it seems little appears to have changed since the seventeenth century in the ways in which black women and men continue to be represented and the positioning of black and white peoples, male and female. This history forms part of all of our cultural heritage. It informs the ways in which we (white and black, men and women) relate to each other in contemporary Britain. As Donna, a 29-year-old black woman[5] user of mental health services voiced in a recent interview[6] with me:

that's all our fears, black, white or whatever, of being eliminated
... the system gets you into a fight where it's your fault – it's my fault;
you're stupid; you're okay/ you're superior – I'm inferior ... When
you've been told from when you're small like it is you and everything
out there's okay – well you think everything's okay. But it's not okay.
How can it be okay if something is based on lies? You try to get rid
of a particular 'race' saying that they've got no culture, no history –
they don't exist – I think I've got every right to be angry.

In the context of this cultural heritage, we must now consider how this shapes, and is shaped by, the (statistical) representation of black women within the statutory health service.

The changing National Health Service

The government has identified two main areas to be addressed in relation to inequities experienced by black peoples: their employment position across all NHS structures (MMd/MAS update, 1993) and their general under-representation as users of a range of services (e.g. Department of Health, 1993b). In particular, the government has emphasized that 'service provision should be sensitive to the local situation whereby the local demographic composition should be statistically reflected in its employment policies and that any differences in service provision for different groups are accounted for' (Department of Health, 1993a: p. 35). Changes in these areas could counter the conception of the health service as a predominantly white institution which does not value, understand, or have the skills required to work with black peoples and which could be the key to improving voluntary access to the services (Nadirshaw, 1993; Department of Health, 1993b; NHS Task Force, 1994a).

One difficulty in assessing the present position of black women in relation to mental health services is the lack of systematic, comprehensive and comparable data available in relation to categories of 'race' and 'gender' (Sayal, 1990). This both contributes to and reflects the invisibility of black women and their needs as users or providers of services. Moreover, the validity of any data collected, whether grounded in equal opportunities monitoring or clinical and epidemiological research, has been variously challenged. Criticisms include that systems in place (of 'ethnic' and equal opportunities monitoring) typically adopt homogeneous and static concepts of identity which obscure the diverse and dynamic aspects of self-definitions; conflate concepts of 'race' with 'ethnicity' and 'culture'; and reify 'race' rather than acknowledge its social and political origins and significance (Cohen, 1988; Webb-Johnson, 1991; Sashidharan and Francis, 1993). Hence, as the following sections will indicate, the specific positions of black women are at times rendered invisible.

Policy makers/administrators of service provision

Since 1989 the primary responsibility for responding to the British nation's health needs has been devolved to a more regional/district 'local' level in order to facilitate responsiveness to the needs of the immediate population to be served by particular institutions (NHS Task Force, 1994b). This 'local' level has included the boards of Regional Health Authorities, Special Health Authorities, National Heath Service Trusts and Family Health Service Authorities, in collaboration with the voluntary sector. Criteria for membership of these boards (comprising chairs, executive and non-executive members) is dependent, for example, on decisions by the Secretary of State, existing institutional positions (e.g. the automatic inclusion of hospital managers, medical and finance directors on particular boards) and personal contributions to the effective management of, for example, hospitals and not for any interest group they might represent (Secretary of State, 1989). Since black women are concentrated at the lower levels of a gender-segregated labour market (Brah, 1991) and over the decades have engaged in officially 'low profile' community activism and support for women (Griffin, 1995) such criteria are likely to operate against the identification of black women as objectively 'suitable' for such positions.

Indeed, Hunt (1994) in reviewing the composition of the boards, reported that the chairs and non-executive members were overwhelmingly white (figures ranged from 100 per cent to 97 per cent on the data available at the time), although no analysis of 'gender' was proffered. In general it seems that few representatives from the voluntary sector (where black peoples are characteristically situated and whose projects are often subject to precarious and short-term funding) are involved in the decision-making processes (McIntyre, 1994). Moreover, where representatives of local black communities are consulted, the finding that black women can experience difficulty in having their interests recognized by male representatives further renders black women invisible (Griffin, 1995). Some authors have also illuminated how even where 'minority' group members such as black peoples and/or women are included in the policy-making arenas, power can be employed by dominant groups to ensure that any changes in the *status quo* are those that can be easily incorporated into the existing framework through, for example, non-decision-making processes (Marchbank, 1994) or 'psychological lynching' (Torkington, 1991).

To date, the devolvement of responsibility to the 'local' level appears to have effected little change. As Rogers, Pitgrim and Lacey (1993) point out, 'local' policy statements appear to reflect the same broad generalized statements issued nationally by the Department of Health. In sum, this suggests that black peoples in general, but black women in particular, are unlikely to figure and are likely to remain largely invisible at key managerial and decision-making levels within the NHS.

Providers of services

Although the NHS employs more black peoples than most organizations they (particularly African–Caribbeans) tend to be be overrepresented in ancilliary services and nursing fields (Yeboah, 1988). Studies exploring acceptance rates for training and the commitment to equal opportunities within medicine, psychiatry, (clinical) psychology, psychotherapy and NHS Health Authorities reveal the continuing systematic exclusion/underrepresentation of black peoples and/or the lack of the development and implementation of formal written policies and monitoring (Bhate, 1987; Bender and Richardson, 1990; Mapstone and Davey, 1990; Gordon, 1993; Ward, 1993; Roth and Leiper, 1995). For example, during the 1950s and 1960s with the growing NHS demands, people of Asian origins who trained outside Britain were employed as general practitioners and psychiatrists. However, they have found themselves channelled into lower status positions within medicine, less likely to find permanent positions and consistently having to wait longer for promotion relative to their equally qualified white peers (Littlewood and Lipsedge, 1989; Ward, 1993). As the demands for such practitioners have reduced, so have the acceptance rates for both training and posts – particularly for British-born black peoples (Bhate, 1987; Yeboah, 1988).

Within (clinical) psychology, the position is no better with the numbers of black and Asian psychologists in general, 'so small as to not constitute a power base at all' (Mapstone and Davey, 1990, p. 387). Moreover the possession of an undergraduate degree in psychology is a prerequisite for acceptance for clinical psychology training and as such is subject to all the structural exclusions of the education system. The finding by Bender and Richardson (1990) that between 1978 and 1984 only 4.4 per cent of successful applicants to clinical psychology training courses were of African–Caribbean and/or Indian origins has not improved 10 years on. Of the 1994 cohort of trainees in clinical psychology, only five (2.3 per cent) of 218 successful applicants were of African (one) Caribbean (one) and Indian (three) origins (gender not known): Aitken (in progress). This falls below Bender and Richardson's figures, the 1991 OPCS national population composition (4 per cent) and very likely the demographic composition of the local community (depending on how the notion of 'community' is operationalized) in which particular training/practising institutions are located. When we consider how the findings on 'race' intersect with the general finding that women are concentrated at the lower levels of the profession (Nicolson, 1992), the position for black women again looks particularly bleak.

Even if increased statistical representation of black peoples across mental health professions were to occur, Eurocentric, as well as heterosexist and sexist, theories and practices legitimated by their assumed scientific underpinnings predominate within training (MacCarthy, 1988; Fernando, 1993a; Nadirshaw, 1993). The dissemination of research findings on 'race' differences tend to render black peoples visible only in the 'exotic', or the more pathological categories of mental illness, such as schizophrenia, as contained within the DSM and ICD[7] classification systems for 'mental illness' (Littlewood and Lipsedge, 1989; Ahmad, 1993; Fernando, 1993a, 1993b; Sashidharan and Francis, 1993). As a number of authors have illuminated, such categorization of black peoples might be more appropriately understood as the power of mental health disciplines to pathologize both black peoples' resistance to forms of social control (see e.g. Black Health Workers and Patient Group, 1983) or alternatively as instances of conforming to the ascribed or projected activities which have been constructed for them by white 'scientists'.

Although as students, practitioners and/or researchers we might be encouraged to follow up alternative models and theories in our leisure time, the low (and selective) profile of 'race' and 'ethnic' issues within the central programme of any training course and institution confirms their marginal status. By implication we are expected to internalize the existing and presented frameworks and to apply them in practice. Thus structures are in place which facilitate conformity to existing professional or organizational norms rather than the identification of, resistance against and challenge to oppressive assumptions and practices (which would be at the likely risk of jeopardizing employment, career and funding prospects).

Psychology and psychiatry are underpinned by theories, models and practices which promote the individualization of social distress and social issues and which obscure the wider social, economic and political contexts within which people's experiences are grounded (Marshall, 1988). Users of mental health services may employ strategies of resistance to counter the interrelated effects of racism and sexism both within and outside of the mental health services, such as 'failure to attend' or refusal to take medication. As health professionals, we should be aware how we may unquestioningly (intentionally or unintentionally – see e.g. Ridley, 1995) use our 'expertise' to 'objectively' counter-label such strategies as, for example, non-engagement or non-compliance. Explanations grounded in beliefs of non-compliance may act to confirm to professionals that particular categories of clients are not appropriately 'psychologically-minded' to receive a range of therapies which lie outside non-directive or medicalized forms; whereas non-compliance may confirm that certain categories of peoples are not 'rational' enough to self-medicate, thus legitimizing the use of depots.[8]

Users of services

The perpetuation of historical representations of the inherent genetic–biological/cultural predisposition of black peoples as, for example, dangerous and uncontrollable, intellectually inferior and vulnerable to more serious categories of mental illness is reflected and shaped by their numerical overrepresentation in the involuntary referral routes into mental health services (Littlewood and Lipsedge, 1989; Browne, 1990; Sayal, 1990; Fernando, 1993b). By contrast, interpretations of their more general numerical underrepresentation as (voluntary) users of a range of statutory mental health services similarly problematizes them. Explanations are grounded in assumptions about their lack of reasoning and/or emotional capacity to experience a range of distress, propensity to somatize rather than psychologize their distress, repressive family/religious cultures, a lack of willingness to integrate into wider society and language difficulties. The impact of the possible racist and sexist, or appropriateness of assumptions, models, practices or structures within wider society, disciplines of psychiatry or psychology or within the NHS are rarely considered (Littlewood and Lipsedge, 1989). When issues relating to racism are discussed (Thomas *et al.*, 1993), differences between the rates of diagnosis between different categories of black peoples may be interpreted as not producing clear-cut evidence for the role of racism (rather than as indicating different racialized and racist practices).

In terms of current political agendas, black women have become visible in the *Health of the Nation* targets, although in limited areas. Thus women born outside of Britain and 'Asian' women (particularly of potential marriageable age) have been identified as particularly at risk of self-harm (Department of Health, 1993a). This not only problematizes 'race' and 'place of birth' (ignoring how experiences may be shaped by gender and class specificities since being in Britain), but also confirms a representation of families/cultures of peoples of Asian origins as especially repressive for women (as also identified by the white colonizers of the early twentieth century – see e.g. Ware, 1992). What this obscures is the role of lack of societal resources and services generally available to Asian women (based on the misassumption that Asian families 'prefer to look after their own') and the role of racism within wider society (Webb-Johnson, 1991; Griffin, 1995).

Further, the experiences of black women have been rendered largely invisible in an area which has provoked the greatest criticism of the mental health services: the overrepresentation of black peoples in first and/or (re)admissions under the various sections of the Mental Health Act (1983) and the association with diagnoses of schizophrenia. Significantly, both these reflect the interrelated workings of the police and psychiatric systems (Littlewood and Lipsedge, 1989; Browne, 1990; Fernando, 1993b; Ratna and Wheeler, 1994). Although the rates identified vary (depending on how 'race' is constructed), research suggests that African–Caribbean and Asian groups are more likely than their white peers to experience involuntary admissions and be diagnosed with schizophrenia and that British-born black peoples characteristically experience the highest rates. However, typically such studies (because 'ethnic' monitoring data is not available, or the numbers are small, or there are no statistically significant differences between the genders) 'collapse' women and men into a single category. Such analyses effectively render women invisible and obscure the fact that the common stereotypic representation of the threatening black male is not supported. Nevertheless, some work reports that black women are overrepresented, comprising up to half of the sectionings, and that their behaviour could in any case be described as disruptive rather than dangerous (Browne, 1990; Sayal, 1990; Ratna and Wheeler, 1994). Torkington's (1991) account of the experience of a black woman who, after initially requesting a voluntary referral subsequently found herself positioned as requiring sectioning when she attempted to leave, may be indicative.

The advent of care in the community policies and the increasing promotion of the self-regulation of behaviours (through the use of self-help groups and literature and the widespread availability and use of medication to ward off relapse) has been identified as having particular implications for women. There is much evidence that the burden of community care falls on the women users of mental health services and/or women carers, yet the distribution of state-provided resources are shaped by stereotypical gendered and racialized assumptions of deservingness of support (Smith, 1991) – assumptions such as: women are 'natural' carers; Asian families want to look after their own; African–Caribbean women may see offers of services as too interventionist. All these work to reduce the likelihood of/arguments for support being offered (Webb-Johnson, 1991; Smith, 1991; Wheeler, 1994).

In the two years of my clinical psychology training, I have met black and white women users of our services, whose 'treatment careers' have spanned one to 25 years. Some of the women are very much aware that medication has been promoted as enabling them to stay within their families to undertake prescribed 'caring' roles. Yet they find themselves struggling to counter the consequent experience of disempowerment (associated with the particular diagnosis) within their various communities, as well as the consequences some medications have had on their ability to maintain the 'standards' of behaviour and care-giving expected. When they have 'failed' to cope (or are perceived by others as failing) with their own or others' distress and manifest 'unacceptable behaviour' (such as showing anger or resisting medication), some have found that they themselves have been blamed for not voluntarily accessing services earlier and not complying with medication regimens. They are held responsible for the coercive forms of treatment they subsequently receive.

Conclusion

In attempting to make visible some of the issues which may be associated with the representation and construction of black women and the implications for black women's positions in relation to mental health issues, I have been very much aware that throughout this chapter black women have surfaced only to disappear a paragraph later. I would argue that this reflects the poverty of conceptual formulation and research. While some work challenges the incoherence and instability of representations and categories of black women at the level of cultural assumptions, these are nevertheless realized (produced and performed) within professional/academic structures both within, and out-side, the NHS. This instability of categories as produced by, and through, the practices of regulation and resistance can be regarded as a political resource. For example, when visible as a category, black women have found themselves pathologized as women or as black; when invisible as a category they are still pathologized for their alleged 'lack' of resistance either to 'femininity' or to 'racism'. It is no wonder that black women may feel obliged to choose between gender and 'race' identifications. Thus one challenge for mental health services is to theorize the relations between 'race' and gender as intersecting rather than additive and to treat such categories as self-defined rather than imposing (and thus further institutionalizing) racialized and genderized identities.

In practical terms, whether the proposed changes within the NHS will materially affect the experiences of black women in their future positioning as users or providers of mental health service provision seems doubtful, unless there is increased visibility and depathologization of black women and their experiences and needs. This necessitates the review and explicit (rather than implicit in the name of 'science') politicization of assumptions and practices, particularly across the disciplines and professions associated with the pro-vision of mental health services. Moreover, a radical reform of equal opportunities legislation is needed to shift the emphasis away from simply generating (generalized) policies to evaluating the effects of such policies on people's lived experiences.

For those of us who may feel that, as individuals, we have relatively little power to effect change, I would argue that there are sites of resistance avail-able to us all. For myself, I can look to my relatively privileged position as a white woman training to become an 'officially accredited provider' of clinical psychology services. I believe that part of my role is to attempt to use (and question) this privilege to identify and challenge personal, professional, insti-tutional and ideological assumptions and practices that obscure the disadvan-tages and discriminations experienced by, for example, black women and to try to work with and for black women. In Donna's words: 'all we can do as human beings is try.'

Acknowledgments

I should like to acknowledge all the women and men engaged in struggles for survival and resistance whom I have heard about, read about, met or shared experiences with, and to acknowledge those who still remain largely invisible when 'resources' come to be 'officially distributed'. Over the years, many people have also variously challenged and/or supported my personal and professional assumptions and practices and, although it has sometimes been difficult for me to hear and accept, I hope I can continue to be open to experiencing and learning from this ongoing process. All these people have in some way contributed to the production of this chapter. Finally, I would specifically like to thank Donna who has trusted me to convey her words; to Erica for suggesting to the other co-authors that I be given the opportunity to participate in this collaborative project; and to all the co-authors for their warm welcome, support and constructive comments on my writings.

Notes

1 It is beyond the scope of the present chapter to review the debates about the appropriateness of the interchangeable use of the terms 'race', 'ethnicity', 'culture' and 'nationality'; readers are referred to, for example, Booth (1988); Ramazanoglu (1989); Donald and Rattansi (1992).
2 Readers requiring the specific references can obtain them from the British Psychological Society.
3 See also the classic Broverman *et al.* (1970) study which demonstrated how women are 'naturally pathologized' when compared to males in judgements of mental health.
4 Involuntary referrals/compulsory admissions into acute psychiatric services are made under various sections of the Mental Health Act (e.g. 1983) and may initially involve the police (if a person is found in a public place and judged to be in need of care and attention), family members, etc. Depending on the referral route, a section order is typically based on the clinical judgement of a medical doctor (experienced in mental health practice) and, if a second opinion is necessary, also by an approved social worker (qualified in mental health service provision). The period of compulsory detainment may vary, as may the review period, and is dependent on the section under which a person is detained.
5 This is 'Donna's' choice of pseudonym and present (political) self-definition.
6 This work forms part of a larger interview project which aims to explore and contextualize the 'treatment careers' of a small number of women of African–Caribbean and Asian origins who are referred to clinical psychology services and to compare their perceptions with those of the referrer and therapist.
7 In Britain, researchers characteristically use the *Diagnostic and Statistical Manual of Mental Disorders* (DSM) – now in its fourth edition – devised by the American Psychiatric Association (APA). Practice psychiatrists tend to use the *International Classification of Diseases* (ICD) – now in its tenth edition – a worldwide system which incorporates both physical and mental 'diseases and disorders' and is devised by the World Health Organization (WHO). The two organizations are increasingly working more closely together in developing and refining their classifications to ensure greater compatability between the two systems.

8 These take the form of injections characteristically administered by appropriately qualified health professionals, which release 'medication' into the
body over a period of weeks and months, thus obviating reliance on the oral
consumption of medication.

Chapter 6

Special women, special places:
Women and high security mental hospitals

Sam Warner

This chapter takes as its site of interrogation women and high security mental hospitals, or 'special' hospitals as they are euphemistically called in Britain. In this chapter we look at how 'woman' is constructed through discourses around madness, criminality and dangerousness and further interpolated through an emerging story of child sexual abuse. We explore how notions of essentialized femininity are both produced and are productive in defining what is normal and abnormal female behaviour and how this process is naturalized so that disposal of these particular women is achieved with little cultural comment or resistance. We address how these women are further defined by their experiences of sexual abuse and the reproduction of normalizing discourses in the practices defining these institutions. Finally, we open out the discussion of resistance to offer some analysis of the limitations of the identities in which these women are written.

Psychological practices, therefore, form the focus of this chapter; not, or not only as some 'expert' knowledge that is dispensed or withheld, but as a resource of 'common sense'. We show how supposed 'truths' of human psychology are used to inform regulatory practices and how the production of such 'truths' is concealed within the very practices they are used to justify. In order to emphasize the discursive production of these 'truths' we use terms such as fictions and stories. These exemplify and sometimes conflict with broader meta-narratives or social themes – thus intimating sites of both more insidious regulation and of possible resistances. Similarly, to emphasize the textual process of producing this chapter, 'we' functions as the fictional author.

We argue that underlying the meta-narratives of criminality, madness and dangerousness are assumptions also associated with normative understandings of child sexual abuse and that these accounts are both gendered and gendering. So while 'woman' as a category may occupy different discursive locations, within this particular articulation a limitation of role is enforced. Once named as 'woman' in this particular story of incarceration (a female special hospital patient), this name serves as the prediscursive right to enact regulation against transgression. Femininity, then, is enforced via institutions and the practices which give rise to them. The aim here is to focus on the particular – on some of those on the margins of femininity. These women are not so much our 'other', but rather what we might become should we transgress cultural stereotypes too much.

In this chapter we are concerned with the practices of disposing of this particular group of women. But more than this, we aim to articulate how this particular gendered identity, while being on the margins of femininity, is also produced through the same normative narratives. As such we are not interested in discovering the 'truth' of femininity, but why certain knowledges that are presented as truths subjugate other knowledges; why some stories become so powerful and readily available that they function as truths. We will not, therefore, address the origin of these institutions or the stories which hail them, but rather focus on the interplay of these stories as they are enacted now.

In framing this project we borrow from Foucault (1977a, 1992) and Butler (1990b, 1993b). We understand power as always immanent in the construction of truth. 'There is no "outside" to power and no male possession of power' (Bailey, 1993, p. 117). Discourses become institutionalized as practices through which power is deployed. Truth, then, is produced rather than revealed. Hence we can interrogate how femininity is produced in culture and how a particular female subject is interpolated within these particular settings. We can begin to explore how men and women are differentially produced within discourse. This calls for a more complex reading of power. As Foucault (1977a, pp. 26–7) suggests:

> power is exercised rather than possessed; it is not a 'privilege', acquired or preserved, of the dominant class, but the overall effect of its strategic positions – an effect that is manifest and sometimes extended by those who are dominated. Furthermore, this power is not exercised simply as an obligation or prohibition on those who 'do not have it'; it invests them, is transmitted by them and through them; it exerts pressure on them, just as they themselves, in their struggle against it, resist the grip it has on them.

'Being a woman' is not the source of action, but in action 'woman' is produced. In this sense bodies are given the fiction of stability, while in the same moment, as 'woman' is not a unitary category, this 'inevitably generates multiple refusals to accept the category' (Butler, 1990b, p. 4). Hence, there is an inevitable link between regulation and resistance. As Bordo (1992, p. 93) notes, while history may appear as a logical progression, like Foucault, she suggests that there is no need to invoke an agency to invent aims and strategies. Moreover, while power relations involve the domination of one group or another, the dominators are not always in control and sometimes it is the dominated who extend and advance the situation themselves. Hence, power is a 'generative force as well as a restrictive opportunity' (Bell, 1993, p. 109).

Sam Warner

Raising questions and disrupting the process

Admission to a maximum security mental hospital, of which there are three in England (Ashworth, Broadmoor and Rampton) is achieved in relation to three related criteria: the patient must be deemed to possess a treatable mental disorder; to be a danger to society or, if not society, then themselves; and, usually, they will have committed a criminal offence which has brought them to the attention of the authorities. Some patients will come directly from other mental institutions when they can no longer 'cope' with the patient, but usually an index offence, albeit small, will have been committed. There are currently about 300 women patients in British special hospitals, who make up less than 20 per cent of the population, aged between 18 years to 55 plus (Reed Report, 1994). Patients in special hospitals are always compulsorily detained under the Mental Health Act (1983), often without a time limit.

Three meta-narratives of madness, criminality and dangerousness are invoked in defining these women and their treatment. Underlying these narratives are psychological fictions which, through their incorporation within the overarching truisms of madness and criminality, serve to reproduce and regulate behaviour. Such knowledges, then, are used to police the boundaries between abnormality and normality.

Through these stories identity is given the fiction of stability. Identity is cited as the basis on which judgements are made, rather than through which identity is produced and reproduced. As stable subjects, decisions can be made about them: decisions which constrain and exclude them from the rest of society. These identities then serve to legitimate action and intervention. We argue, therefore, that the notion of 'identity' is politically critical because once identity is produced the exclusionary practices which construct identity are rendered invisible by a juridical system which takes identity as foundational. So, like Butler (1990b, pp. 5–6), we believe, 'The task is to formulate within this constituted frame a critique of the categories of identity that contemporary juridical structures engender, naturalise, and immobilise.' The question therefore arises: if gender is the regulation of attributes, what particular attributes are called into being in the process of producing these 'special' women?

Getting there: discursive routes to incarceration

Madness

Madness is a particularly potent aspect of the cultural economy which serves to prescribe behaviour and values. It is beyond the scope of this chapter to delve into all its variability. Here we are primarily interested in some of its gendered assumptions and gendering effects, as they are played out within medico-legal discourse and practices. At the most parsimonious level, madness is counterpoised to reason and may be recognized as the presence of the inappropriate. A corollary of this is that dominant cultural inscriptions of madness rely on normalizing fictions which are presented as truths. One pervasive and relevant truth is of discrete subjectivities of male and female.

Various feminist critiques have been offered in order to understand women's madness (see Chapter 4 for a critique of feminist psychotherapy). For Chesler (1972), madness is understood in terms of the devalued female role. As Russell (1995, p. 113) notes, 'Mere unhappiness in one's role does not constitute madness, but alienation from or rejection of one's role does.' It is not just a 'lack' of power and limitation of roles of rejection, however, but that through the gendering process women come to embody madness. So, as Ussher (1991, pp. 11–12), argues:

> 'Madness' acts as a signifier which positions women as ill, as outside, as pathological, as somehow second-rate – the second sex . . . Thus, the discursive practices which create the concept of madness mark it as fearful, as individual, as invariably feminine, as sickness.

Feminist theorists refer to history to emphasize both the social construction of women's madness and the resilience of gendered inequality in the reproduction and stability of these relationships (Spender, 1994). We agree that 'woman' occupies a specifically delineated role in relation to madness. However, like Allen (1987, p. 11) we are aware that such an analysis is in danger of being overinclusive:

> According to this model, the basis of psychiatrisation of female offenders is either their 'acting out' of the prescribed female role or their rejection of some or all aspects of it. Put these two categories together and they cover the entire field, embracing all female offenders, if not the entire population of women.

We argue, therefore, that while madness cannot be totally reduced to the effects of patriarchy nor that the ascription of madness and the effects of this is predictable and necessarily bad, women are positioned centrally in relation to discourses over madness. We are not interested in proving or disproving madness, nor in reifying patriarchy – but in how power–knowledge systems produce subjects. Whatever madness is, one thing we can say is that women 'have' more of it or are more frequently defined in relation to it then men. So, for example, women are more likely to be compulsorily detained in psychiatric wards than are men (Barnes and Maple, 1992, p. 139). More specifically, proportionately more women than men are diverted from the criminal system into special hospitals. This leads Lloyd (1991, p. 36) to argue that:

> the fact that there are proportionately more women than men in Specials is a reflection of two things: the views of psychiatrists and

those within the criminal justice system as to what is appropriate behaviour for women, and the feeling that women are not necessarily in control of their actions and therefore need care.

Hence the 'usefulness' of dumping these non-women in special hospitals – and, once dumped, women will spend proportionately far longer, for often less serious offences than men (Stevenson, 1990). Defining and classifying these women has the dual effect of defining the norm for the rest of us. It is in relation to this norm that some of us come to know ourselves as valid or disqualified as the approximation of woman.

Medico-legal discourses and practices are therefore saturated with the pervasiveness of women's madness. So how does this saturation lead to women being diverted from criminal into medical contexts and what kind of female subject is produced? Notions of femininity as victim are reified and are produced within medico-legal stories as well as feminist ones. Woman is variously victim of biology – woman *qua* woman (medico-legal) or victim of patriarchy (feminism).

Badness

At the heart of the law in Britain is the notion of the 'reasonable man'. This is in relation to criminal culpability: would a 'reasonable man' do the same in similar circumstances? Even before we add the additional fiction of madness, gendering has begun. The notion of a 'reasonable man' was extended in the law to include the particular age and sex of the defendant (Allen, 1987, p. 23) – but with few actual provisions for sex difference in the law. Infanticide has been a notable exception. The only other obvious area where men and women are explicitly differentiated is where the presence of premenstrual syndrome has been used as a legal defence. So where gender specific stories are used, they further produce woman as victim: women's biology is somehow inherently sick, pathological and mad. Concomitantly, as Worrall argues (1990, p. 97), there is 'a socio-legal belief in the fundamental "normality" of *man*'. She goes on to argue that concessions are made 'to those defendants who suffer the misfortune of being *non-male*'.

What are these concessions? Somehow, while it is acceptable for men to be bad, similarly, as it is deemed unfeminine to be bad, there is a rush to apply the label of madness to women law-breakers. Lloyd (1991) notes that women make up 4 per cent of the prison population, but 20 per cent of patients in special hospitals. Kennedy (1993, p. 23) indicates the deeper social investments in containing women's badness as madness:

> Because we feel differently about women committing crime, we go to great lengths to avoid defining them as criminal, preferring the idea that they have emotional problems; they are mad rather than bad.

Allen (1987) further notes that psychiatric involvement at the courts serves to liberalize the medicalization of female offenders and to restrict medical involvement with males. So the courts treat women as more mad than bad. Collier and Dibblin (1990) note that a woman appearing in the criminal courts is twice as likely to be sent for psychiatric treatment as a man. They quote a Broadmoor psychiatrist, Dr Mezey, who says if a woman has transgressed against the law and the code of feminine docility, passivity and gentility:

> She may be regarded as doubly bad, doubly evil, and put into prison for a long time or, if she is not bad, therefore she must be very, very mad and in need of psychiatric treatment in high security.

Hence, within dominant discourses of femininity, it is easier to view women who deviate as mad rather than address the irrationality of these codes. Where women have transgressed femininity and also escaped psychiatrization, they may be deemed 'purely bad'. If this is the case then no allowances are forthcoming, as is the case with Myra Hindley who, with her partner, Ian Brady, was responsible for the abuse and murder of a number of children in the early 1960s. So while the coupling of madness and women within the law is pervasive, it is not entirely exclusive.

The fiction of woman as mad within the law is powerfully productive in interpreting behaviour such that as women are already associated with being 'mad', little is needed to crystallize this label. Similar events and behaviour are interpreted differently according to gender. Different criteria are used to judge men and women within the same categories of criminal/legal culpability, pathology and clinical need (Allen, 1987). So although the typical construction of the female mentally disordered person is often less than a disordered male and would militate against psychiatric disposal, in fact it operates in reverse. This is not because she is a woman, but rather her gender is constructed as such throughout this process. Men and women are judged against different sets of criteria, which thereby construct gender differences through this process in a circular and confirmatory way. So as Worrall (1990, p. 113) points out:

> By invoking the female domination of the official statistics of mental illness to demonstrate that even 'normal' women are prone to mental instability, those women who deviate from normal gender expectations by breaking the law are viewed as doubly prone to such instability.

Moreover, because of the pervasiveness of feminine madness, specific recognition of women is rendered difficult. Allen (1987) noted that most descriptions offered to her of 'mentally disordered offenders' were male and was told that few women came into the system. However, the descriptions she looked at offered by professionals of women law-breakers who behaved in the same way as 'mad' male offenders were recorded as normal or not 'mad'.

At the same time so-called normal (male) behaviours are used to pathologize women offenders. Psychopathic personality disorder is a legal term which may be used to divert defendants into medical, rather than criminal, fictions. Women are one-and-a-half times more likely than men to be diagnosed as suffering from a psychopathic disorder (Lloyd, 1991) – though interestingly the cultural available image of the psychopath is a (white) man (see Parker *et al.*, 1995). Regarding some of the so-called clinical evidence for psychopathy Allen (1987, p. 80) notes:

> Educational maladjustment, disorderly behaviour, lack of emotional ties, illicit drug use and sexual activity outside marriage: all of these breach the expectation of conventional femininity, and in young women provide evidence that she is a psychopath. In a male, however, they may be acknowledged as socially deviant, but they are still consistent with the expectations of masculine normality, and are therefore treated as no more than ordinary delinquency.

As can be seen, the construction of woman as mad is not unidirectional, but paradoxical. The process of pathologization of woman in the law is not to defeminize her, but rather to account for her apparent lack of femininity as being hidden under the cloak of madness. Hence, the assertion of femininity can be used to confirm her criminal culpability *and* to divert her into medical contexts. Furthermore, when additional stories such as 'race' are told, the end result of a feminizing story becomes even more unstable. Black women are overrepresented among women in prison (Lloyd, 1995, p. 136), it is argued, because they transgress femininity. Thus to be constructed as black and female is to be more bad than mad. This is precisely the same reason why more women, generally, are pathologized. (The relationship between race, gender and mental health was explored further in Chapter 5.)

Woman as victim is crystallized in the law's tactics of pathologization. As she is 'troubled', 'mad', 'sick' she is not responsible for her crimes and so should be diverted from systems of punishment into systems of treatment. And while incarceration in secure mental hospitals may be perceived as punishment, it is dressed up in the language of need and treatability which then legitimizes incarceration (see Chapter 7 for a related discussion on the regulation of 'special need' children). The crime is storied as a 'cry for help' in which her victim status is confirmed – she is not culpable but she will be punished/ locked up/ pathologized.

> I've been away from home since I was 13 years old. The first time it was to remand home, then hospital, then children's homes and then prisons. I was always doing wrong things to try and make people care. It was a kind of cry for help. (Diane, RSU (Regional Secure Unit), *WISH* (Women in Special Hospitals) *Newsletter*, 1994, p. 7)

Dangerousness

The final discourse in this particular trinity is that of dangerousness. While women may be more pathological than men in medico-legal stories, it is the fiction of dangerousness which gives the final justification for incarceration in institutions of maximum security. Danger may be in terms of the risk posed to 'the public' or the risk posed to the self. As can be seen from the differential diagnosis of psychopathic disorder, constituent behaviours need be much less extreme for women than for men. But despite this she may still be deemed 'in need' of maximum security. Returning to an earlier point, if women are essentialized as possessing a naturally dangerous body, what raises these women above the bounds of 'ordinary femininity'?

Certainly some women in special hospitals have acted in a dangerous manner: a significant number of women fire-set and so constitute a danger to property. However, the coupling of danger and women usually refers to her danger to herself: in terms of self-harm and/or her self-neglect. This self-harm may go beyond what staff in other institutions can deal with or watch. Indeed, while some of the women who end up in special hospitals may represent a danger to others, the vast majority of them self-harm to an extreme degree. But again the danger to herself may not necessarily be extreme. For example, Shepperd (1990) quotes a member of staff accounting for restricting the liberty of one female patient: 'In the past she has been at risk of going out late and chatting up men. It hasn't happened so far, but on past performance I expect it would.'

Medico-legal discourses, then, both rely on and reproduce notions of essentialized femininity within which all women are constructed. Even those women who might be said to be on the margins of dominant female identity are nevertheless judged and reproduced in relation to this. Normative assumptions underlie the grand narratives of madness, criminality and dangerousness which serve to engender subjectivity and to particularize femininity as passive, as victim. So although practices and knowledges construct 'woman' generally, this does not necessarily result in a clear path through the courts to special hospitals – although for some women their particular storying and invocation of the above fictions means that this is where they end up.

Being there – special/invisible/(feminine)

Mental asylums rarely offer asylum. Both their calculated and their haphazard brutality mirrors the brutality of 'outside' society. The 'scandals' about them that periodically surface in the media are like all atrocities – only everyday events writ large. Madness – as a label or reality – is not conceived of as divine, prophetic, or useful. It is perceived as (and often further shaped into) a shameful and menacing disease, from whose spiteful and exhausting eloquence society must be protected . . . At their worst, mental asylums are families bureaucratized: the degradation and disenfranchisement of self, experienced by the biologically owned child (patient, woman), takes place in the anonymous and therefore guiltless embrace of strange fathers and mothers. In general psychiatric wards and state hospitals, 'therapy', privacy and self-determination are all either minimal or forbidden . . . Mental patients are somehow less 'human' than either medical patients or criminals. They are, after all, 'crazy'. (Chesler, 1972, pp. 34–5)

Chesler wrote the above of mental institutions in America in 1972 but her account still resonates with special hospitals today. But special hospitals are not just about the disenfranchisement and production of the 'mad', they are also productive of the 'bad'. So while the Reed Report (1994, annex 2) notes that 'the special hospitals are very clearly hospitals and not prisons', it goes on to note that they occupy a space somewhere in between criminal and mental health systems:

They are different from prisons because they exist to treat patients, and not merely to contain them and their philosophy and culture must be that of the National Health Service. They are different from other psychiatric hospitals and regional secure units by reason of their heightened security measures . . . The special hospitals are by definition different and should be seen as different. This calls for a very high order of professionalism from all staff.

This 'professionalism', in the past, has meant that most of the nursing staff have been members of the Prison Officers Association, rather than any of the nursing trade unions which is indicative of the pervasiveness of a discourse of badness, criminality and culpability. Patients are 'specialled', in as much as they are fictionalized at the intersection of all three of the discourses of madness, badness and criminality outlined earlier. They are not just bad or mad but both. And although bad and mad women may be different from bad and mad men, both in their construction and in the judgements made of them, special hospital patients are often conflated within the public gaze such that women as the minority become hidden within the predominant story of mad and bad male patients. So women are invisible as (male) patients and are concealed within the general (male) story. In the public gaze men and women patients are all bad and dangerous in the same way and so the public remain disinterested in their fate. In effect women need to commit less serious offences in order to be perceived as just as dangerous as men.

Special hospitals are also invisible, away from society down leafy roads, somewhere we place people we wish to forget, private and removed. At the same time special hospitals are stories of infamy, housing the most terrible spectres of society: a role call of infamous men from Ian Brady to Peter Sutcliffe. Their dual purpose is to contain and cure; to take away liberty and so function as punishment and to act as change agent to produce Foucault's 'docile bodies' – of which later. These places then function as total institutions, separate from although bound up with the world, continuous and complete in and of themselves. They operate not just as places of exclusion but as technologies of production, of individualization of the gendered subject. They produce and specify a particular 'criminally insane' female.

So, while women remain the predominantly identified patients within mental hospitals generally, they are often invisible within the male society of the special hospitals. This paradox has been recognized and the invisible is in the process of being made visible:

> there are relatively more women in Special hospitals than in prison, but relatively fewer women in Special hospitals than in psychiatric hospitals generally. General psychiatric admission rates for women are higher than for men (including for personality disorders, psychosis generally and drug and alcohol dependency). More widely the needs of women are often poorly catered for by services for mentally disordered offenders which deal mainly with men. (The Reed Report, 1994, p. 29)

The current lack of designated 'women's needs' is reflected in access to, for example, institutional working parties. One woman patient made two attempts to join a working group, where she was the only woman. On both occasions she was removed, after being sexually assaulted by male patients (personal communication, 1990, 1994).

Recent attempts have been made to 'special' the women and provide specialist services. Broadmoor and Ashworth appointed women service managers and Rampton a women's service adviser. Their role was to develop and establish initiatives which would benefit all women patients. But after less than one year the women's service manager at Ashworth was seconded elsewhere and has not been replaced. The adviser at Rampton resigned, also after less than one year in post, saying:

> Hospital Management should stop patting themselves on the back and talking about 'improving services'. It is time they actually do something and this means more than providing pastel wallpaper, knitting classes and talking about market economy. (*WISH Newsletter*, 1994, p. 9)

Special, in this formulation then, equates with normative. Women continue to be defined in passive and yet responsible ways (such that it is possible for a woman to be 'punished' by being removed from the working group in which she was assaulted. She is both victim and seducer). Women patients are both special/visible and under a male cloak/invisible. To be made visible is to be defined and regulated and rendered impotent, as the feminine. Or to be publicly visible, like Beverly Allitt, who killed a number of children while working as a nurse, for example, is to be somehow a 'non-woman' (and most definitely bad). In the following sections we explore how female normalization is achieved in relation to discourses over sexual abuse and sexuality and more generally as the 'female patient'.

Sexing the patient – child sexual abuse, enforced heterosexuality and (sexual) assault

While child sexual abuse and sexual violence have been important fictions in storying special hospitals for some time, it has been a way of storying male patients as abusers: the aforementioned Ian Brady and Peter Sutcliffe are two particularly well-known names. It is only in recent times that child sexual abuse has emerged as both an area of expert knowledge and a story in which to site and hail female patients – and male patients (as victims). Women are both fictionalized as passive victim and as active seducer. This is in relation to the identities mapped out for women, the provision of services and their careers in these services. Since the late 1980s sexual abuse has become part of the storying of women in the narrative of their journey into special hospitals:

> The vast majority of female patients have been seriously sexually abused and been subjected to violence by men in their past. Most of them have been neglected, they have been in and out of care. They have gradually become criminalized, in and out of penal institutions and hospitals and have eventually ended up in Ashworth Hospital having offended. (Dr Gravett, psychiatrist, HMSO, 1992a, p. 229)

Many of the symptoms regularly attributed to having been sexually abused are also written in the symptoms of major psychiatric disorders such as personality disorders (psychopathic, borderline, multiple: see Russell, 1995, for a brief discussion of this), schizophrenia (Friedman and Harrison, 1984), and general psychiatric symptoms and disorders (Pribor and Dinwiddie, 1992). Such 'disorders' are the diagnoses that signify entrance to special hospitals. In particular, younger women are increasingly diagnosed as suffering from personality disorders (Reed Report, 1994).

At the moment of sexual abuse women are interpellated as 'girls', as 'victim' and these identities are reinstituted in the moments of being a special hospital patient. This is evident in the language used. In the Ashworth inquiry (HMSO, 1992a, p. 230) it was noted that:

> Language is an important indicator of attitude. Women in Ashworth are commonly referred to as 'girls'. We heard much evidence that

other more offensive, abusive words are used at times by staff when referring to, and when addressing women – 'slags', 'sluts', 'wops', 'mess-pots'.

This is in addition to other terms which denote fixed and devalued identities, such as a black woman in one special hospital being referred to as 'nig', at a time when British National Party stickers declaring 'white supremacy' and calling for the 'outlawing' of homosexuality could be found on wards, put there by staff (personal experience, 1990).

Yet women are still rendered not responsible (irresponsible?) for their crimes; Barwick (1992) quotes an unnamed ex-patient:

They still don't take me seriously. They made excuses for my crime. I was female, was gay, my background was middle class. So I had to be sick. I couldn't be bad. I wanted to go to prison, do my time, but no.

She was sent to Broadmoor; her offence left an elderly women with 40 stitches in her head. But women are still punished for being women and at the same time inculcated into heterosexuality. Barwick (1992):

Like other women patients, many of whom have been sexually abused as children, she was made, as part of her 'treatment', to 'socialise with men'. In Broadmoor, of course, the supply of eligible men was limited. 'So they placed us in a little disco at 4.30 pm for a nice bit of socialising with a lot of sex offenders.'

Barnes and Potier (1993) offer further examples of this. Indeed, women patients continue to be actually sexually assaulted by male patients (personal communications, 1994). Sexual assault is not only the province of male patients; women's bodies generally are under male domain. Kim Andrews, ex-patient (1990) recalls:

A lot of the time was spent in 'seclusion', naked except for a strong nightdress. I would be attended to by male staff, even to them bringing me a clean sanitary towel and removing the soiled one. I found the whole procedure degrading and despicable; the longer I rotted the more bitter and frustrated I became, and the more volatile my protests became.

Little recognition of how this might feel is evident in this quote from the POA (Prison Officers' Association):

In referring to menstruation and other aspects of women's lives . . . [we] would go further and suggest that male staff show a greater degree of sensitivity in such matters because, perhaps, of their ability as males to be more detached and objective about problems which are essentially female in their origin. (HMSO, 1992a, p. 230)

While it is hoped that since the Ashworth inquiry some changes have been enforced, it is still not long ago that a young woman (with a history of sexual abuse) was forcibly stripped by eight male nurses before being put in seclusion (Stevenson, 1990). Moreover, complaints against staff go largely unheard or are dismissed (Potier, 1993). This is not unsurprising in an institution where 'bad' women (as with 'bad' women generally) are constructed as liars and troublemakers (as well as 'mad'/victim):

The male nursing staff in particular are subjected, not just in Ashworth Hospital but in other hospitals in the country, to allegations which cannot be supported because they did not happen. They are subjected to frequent allegations of matters of a sexual nature and in the majority of cases they do not happen and that is why they are unsupported, because they did not occur. (Mr Barsted, Director of Nursing Services, HMSO, 1992b, p. 82)

The experience of being in a largely male defined environment engenders passivity generally, as one patient poses and answers the questions:

Why is everyone so motiveless? The reason is – that all these occupational activities are male dominated, there being an average eight men to every woman . . . There is a genuine need for us women to be respected and not have to live our lives as brain dead, numb people. That is sadly how the regime of this hospital makes us feel and act. (Anon, Ashworth, *WISH Newsletter*, 1994)

Specifically designated workshops, as suggested earlier, are gender normalizing and uninspiring. Kim, an ex-special hospital patient, quoted by Bedell (1990) notes:

It's not right for women to smash windows. But then half the women I met in Broadmoor had behaved in ways that weren't acceptable for women. They didn't need to be there. The only way to get out is to conform. That means behaving in a ladylike way. They make you wear a skirt and do workshops in knitting, needlework and soft-toy making.

Kennedy (1993) notes that inappropriate behaviour such as being aggressive and/or generally acting inappropriately for their sex gets women into special hospitals. In particular, she argues that lesbians are susceptible to being labelled 'inappropriate'. Normative heterosexuality is not just prescribed at the level of pressure to attend discos with men and pursue 'women's' activities, but is also present in the pressure to wear dresses, make-up and for women to grow their hair and have tattoos removed. Such general practices led Potier (1993, p. 339) to conclude:

> women are dominated, depersonalised, infantilised, and at times physically manhandled. Acceptable behaviour is inculcated by rules which are fossilised as 'custom and practice', overtly restrictive and arbitrarily invoked in the name of security. To date the institution has sanctioned the total invasion and control of every aspect of patient's lives . . . in this the dynamics of abusive histories are re-enacted by the institution which cannot fail to do this.

Women storied within these fictions may occupy the victim role as a necessary, but temporary refuge – if this is the main identity on offer, how else can they get out or exist? Such fictions of feminine passivity and infancy are further reinforced through additional regulatory practices. So in special hospitals women are both mad and bad; they have gone too far beyond the bounds of womanhood and are guilty of being both feminine and not feminine enough. They are responsible victims; what they get they bring on themselves and therefore deserve. The identity hailed by storying sexual abuse is replayed and maintained.

Special/visible – women patients and practices of regulation

Power produces both regulation and resistance which is crystallized in the subject positions or identities which are thus interpellated. As Foucault (1977a, p. 25) argues, 'It is always the body that is at issue – the body and its forces, their utility and their docility, their distribution and their submission.' These bodies become known through their objectification as objects of knowledge. In special hospitals women are categorized, individualized and their every action surveyed.

The power to discipline is written in the Mental Health Act (1983):

> At base, the Mental Health Act defines what may be called mental disorder in our society, and under what circumstances the freedom to seek or disregard treatment may be suspended and the individual obliged to accept medical advice. To be sectioned, therefore, means to have no choice in how some piece of behaviour is to be interpreted and called evidence of mental disorder, no choice in whether to seek help and accept treatment – these decisions, and the sense of autonomy that they engender, are taken out of your hands. (Barnes *et al.*, 1990, p. 12; quoted by Barnes and Maple, 1992, p. 121)

Sam Warner

Foucault's analysis of the panopticon is apposite here (1977a). He noted that the architectual design of modern prisons always rendered the subject open to surveillance and that the fact of being *capable* of being watched is as powerful, in terms of self-regulation, as actual surveillance. Therefore individuals become self-governing. Regulation is institutionalized and becomes localized at the individual. The major effect of the panopticon, then, is 'to induce in the inmate a state of conscious and permanent visibility that assures the automatic functioning of power' (1977a, p. 201). While Foucault was referring to prisons, this resonates with special hospitals:

> Women complain that, like women in prison they are treated like children, that they have no responsibility or control over their everyday lives, essential for their eventual rehabilitation. Every emotion is monitored and commented upon. They are patronised and condescended to. There is no privacy, every aspect of their lives is open to inspection. (Stevenson, 1990)

Although there is 'security' which may come with surveillance and women may be caught within this 'disciplinary gaze', there is no stability:

> Yes, we have security – we are under constant surveillance from cameras as well as staff. We will be locked in our rooms at night. Yet we don't have stability where it matters most. In the past eighteen months the psychiatrist has stayed only three to four months at a time, so decisions don't get made, because they won't until they know the patients and they are gone before this. (Terrie, Broadmoor, *WISH Newsletter*, 1994, p. 19)

Potier (1993; HMSO, 1992a, 1992b) identifies specific techniques of oppression which include seclusion, totalitarian tactics (the promotion of 'top-dogs' and the use of these against other patients) and emotional abuse (relating to inappropriate touching and kissing and the offensive language used). She also identifies techniques of suppression including dropping stages (conditional rights), overmedication, double standards (nurses are routinely offensive, but patients who exhibit such language/behaviour are put on report), divulging confidential information about patients and staff to patients (regarding, for example index offence), the maintenance of disturbance (overtime rewards) and intimidation and dirty tricks. She goes on to argue that as a result of employing such techniques, women try to take the initiative by 'engaging in self-injurious behaviour, eating disorders and, more rarely, non-compliance through open aggression and anger. These latter behaviours usually quickly translate into withdrawal, depression, despair and requests for over-medication' (Potier, 1993, p. 342). This process thus produces Foucault's 'docile bodies'.

However, within special hospitals, the underlying normative assumptions drawn on to produce and maintain women as docile, victim, inwardly as opposed to outwardly aggressive, cannot be totalizing. They prescribe the regulatory ideal, rather than the lived identity of every feminine subject in special hospitals; women do not always self-harm, do continue to define themselves as lesbian and do find their way out. The very fact that such women occupy a space outside the feminine ideal destabilizes the whole concept of identity and in particular that of 'woman'. In Butler's (1990b) terms these women represent 'unintelligible' genders/identities precisely because they fail to conform to cultural norms of intelligibility, while nevertheless being construed in those terms. So not to conform may be to be rendered logically impossible/a failure, but within this complex of positions are the sediments of resistance.

Disrupting identity: women patients and resistance revisited

Resistance to something can also work to reify the structure being resisted, the structure with which it engages. Therefore regulation cannot be unravelled without resistance, or vice versa. Both regulatory fictions and stories of resistance serve to construct femininity. While popular discourses surrounding these particular women may be pejorative, they are not totalizing. There are alternative fictions which occupy the spaces not covered by dominant discourses, which means alternative strategies exist. This is evident in the continuing dialogue between advocates for and critics of special hospitals, from both within and outside the institutions. One particular form of organized resistance can be found in WISH. WISH (Women In Special Hospitals) is a registered charity working on behalf of women in or released from special hospitals, regional secure units and prison psychiatric units. Here the reciprocal relationship between regulation and resistance is manifest; without women in special hospitals WISH could not exist.

While WISH has laudable aims it, like other patients' and prisoners' rights organizations, sometimes draws on the same fictions as the organizations they seek to change. The underlying grip of the binary victim–abuser story running through dominant accounts of women still finds a place within so-called liberatory fictions. WISH, in part, still story women as victims not so much of their biology but of their abused and failed past (it is hard not to). While women in special hospitals have undoubtedly suffered a catalogue of horrors in their lives, should this lead to removing responsibility for crimes committed? Like the liberal advocates of children's rights, advocates for women patients often advocate for the right of women to be good but not bad; to be defined by their advocates rather than the psychiatrists and rather than by their own definition of selfhood. As soon as 'poor' choices (that is to commit offences) are made they are back to being childlike, the victims of circumstance.

There are repeated requests and recommendations for the development of specialist services for women, in particular regarding working with experiences of sexual abuse. But despite this apparently radical-progressive move the system continues to consume these interventions as most still rely on normative assumptions, are individualizing and reproduce gender. So where gender asymmetry is being attacked or there is a wish for change, women are still stuck in the very categories which constrain them. This then is not a simplistic call for treating women and men 'the same'. As Kennedy (1993, p. 31) notes, 'It is no answer to make a simple call for equal treatment. Dealing equally with those who are unequal creates more inequality.' At the same time it is also not enough to argue simply that women's voices should be heard or more fully represented within these institutions, as Showalter (1985) argues.

We need to remain critical of all totalizing theories and therefore need to address how 'women' are restrained and produced through the very structures of power through which emancipation is sought (Butler, 1990b). We need to be critical of any intervention which is based solely on immobilizing gender categories. Otherwise we become stuck in them and limit the possibility for change. In this chapter we have argued that the process of being 'specialed' is not done because some women are women on the margins of femininity, but that the process produces such women as not only marginal but also essentially feminine/passive.

We need to problematize socially instituted gender asymmetry and the assumption of gender as a binary structure. 'Woman' as a category is excluding and normative. We need to disrupt the borders of such notions and fragment what is seen as unitary in order to offer other possibilities. We must be prepared to embrace specificity and learn to attend to the particular. In this sense action needs to be local and policy should reflect flexibility. The very complexity of constructs leads to more possibilities of disrupting gender coherence and therefore regulatory practice; power is generative, not just reproductive. So, however solidified 'women' appear to be, there is always the possibility to offer alternative significations and alternative scripts.

We argue, then, for the subversion of gender categories, rather than to confirm women in them in order to offer the possibility of transformation throughout the 'specializing' process. Our starting point may well be bodies, as Bailey (1993, p. 115) argues:

> Bodies are produced, understood, deployed in the service of certain interests and relations of power. Bodies, thus, are a battleground of interests and power. Foucault's understanding of bodies as the simultaneous source and product of a notion of self allows for strategic redeployment of these embattled bodies.

This is a call for the particularizing of resistance rather than subscription to globalizing strategies, as the means to disrupt the naturalizing of gender and in this the normative assumptions which are used to justify action. There are different levels at which resistance can occur and what is designated as resistance is itself a matter of discursive construction; therefore, we need to continually re-evaluate old strategies. So we must be prepared to determine the setting for a particular event, at a particular time and the methods employed to locate it. As Probyn (1990, p. 182) notes:

> we can nonetheless temper a vision of strict interpelation with the recognition that discourses are negotiated. Individuals live in complex places and differentiate the pull of events. However, if we are to take seriously these relations of place and event, we have to consider the knowledges produced in their interaction.

So the local is a starting point, not the end. And as much as the pull is to rigidity identity and action, this only attests to its instability and therein lies the possibility of change. As Ginger, in *Insiders: Women's Experience of Prisons* (Padel and Stevenson, 1988, p. 124) observes:

> People say that you can't change the system. If that was true we'd still be in Newgate on straw.

Acknowledgments

I am grateful to Ron Blackburn and the research department at Ashworth Hospital for providing the funding for this research project and to Tracy Wilkins, Gill Hall and the rehabilitation service at Ashworth Hospital for their support and enthusiasm.

Chapter 7

Constructing a narrative: Moral discourse and young people's experiences of exclusion

Deb Marks

Introduction

This chapter[1] explores some of the meanings of being excluded from school. It is based on a study of exclusions[2] involving a series of open-ended interviews and group discussions with pupils and a head teacher. The focus of analysis is on exclusion as a lived and socially constituted experience. First, it explores the way exclusion is experienced by pupils and a headteacher. Second, the chapter attempts to make connections between the experience of exclusion and the way accounts of exclusion functioned in the relationship between the researcher and participants in the research. The aim is to offer an analysis of the way exclusion governs the excluded pupil in his (the vast majority of excluded pupils are boys) relationship with the interviewer and with himself. I am using the term 'govern' in the Foucauldian sense (Foucault, 1979a) to refer to an asymmetrical relationship in which one party regulates the conduct and experiences of another 'free agent' .

Before exploring the dynamic context in which exclusion is experienced and accounted for, it is important to note the dramatic escalation in the number of pupils being excluded in recent years (Bennathan, 1993). In response to this increase, there have been a number of studies exploring the relationship between changes in education policy and excluding practices and the possible consequences of exclusion for pupils (Parfrey, 1993). Such questions about why exclusions occur are important, but they do not attend to how the exclusion is accounted for and what it means to pupils and teachers.

Researching experience

The children's rights movement has increasingly proposed that researchers should give children 'a voice' (Cullingford, 1991). They argue that reliance on professional and adult assumptions regarding what pupils feel and do brings with it the danger of commonsense being projected too readily on to complex social phenomena (O'Keeffe, 1994).

The Children Act 1989 indicates that professional and political opinion has accepted the principle that children have a right to be consulted before important decisions are made. However, as Whitney points out, children have far more chance of participating in decisions that affect them 'when they come to the attention of outside agencies' than they have in schools (Whitney, 1993, p. 129). This comment is supported by an Advisory Centre for Education survey (1992) identifying complaints from parents that pupils had not been given the right to attend their exclusion hearing. This is despite research suggesting that when children's views have been solicited (for studies into the efficacy of listening to pupils' views), senior teachers and administrators have been impressed by their 'perception' and 'good sense' (Davie, Phillips and Callely, 1984). It is argued that young people can offer educational professionals a mirror for interrogating their practices.

Alongside greater consideration of young people's voices in social and political contexts, there has been an increasing interest among academic researchers in finding out what young people think (Cullingford, 1991). However, there still remains very little work on the experience of pupils outside mainstream education. More specifically, there has been little work on the experience of pupils who have been excluded and are therefore outside any educational institution. There is, however, some evidence that this situation is beginning to be remedied (Gersch and Nolan, 1994).

However, the whole issue of defining 'rights' is problematic. The human rights discourse sees rights as a property belonging to or conferred upon a person, rather than emerging between people. The discourse of rights is entwined with discourses on responsibility, needs and degrees of dependency. Rights do not exist in the abstract, as the liberal humanist position would claim. What comes to be identified as a right emerges out of specific power relations and forms of knowledge. Thus, endowing young people with the *right* to be heard assumes a particular kind of relationship.

Similarly, researching into people's experience is fraught with epistemological and ontological dilemmas. Social constructionist theory has warned that giving our 'subjects' a 'voice' involves the fantasy that it is possible to have unmediated direct knowledge of experience (such as how it feels to be excluded) (James and Prout, 1990). Derrida (1973) has challenged the phonocentricism implicit in the notion of speech as a direct and immediate form of expression. Giving primacy to interviewees' talk about their experience of exclusion suggests that their speech may refer to themselves as a unified authentic subject. This Cartesian subject, whose self-consciousness acts as guarantor of meaning, is challenged both by versions of psychoanalysis (Althusser, 1971; Frosh, 1987) and discourse analysis (Parker, 1992), which see the subject as being fragmented and constituted within language. Edwards and Middleton (1988) point out that experience and memory are subject to construction and reconstruction over time. Pupils' accounts cannot be seen as final or fixed. Pupils' interpretations of what it means to be excluded do not exist in a static state. Responses are often ambivalent, contradictory and changing.

This reflects both the variability of discourses on exclusion rooted within different pupil cultures (for example, the commonsense understanding among pupils that missing school is desirable exists alongside alternative discourses about the problem of getting into trouble) and the emotional experience of exclusion.

Careful attention to language offers the opportunity of examining how the account of exclusion *functions*. This leads us to analyse accounts in relation to the practices of investigating them. To what extent does 'giving young people a voice' serve to regulate pupils or to create space in which to transform and subvert regulatory control? This chapter does not attempt to see directly into the souls of pupils and the teacher, in order to gain a vantage point from which to understand the experience of exclusion. Rather, the aim here is to explore the relationship between the meanings of exclusion and the context in which they are expressed.

The relationship between an original exclusion and the way pupils talk about it in their interview or discussion group is highly complex. However, this does not invalidate the importance of asking about the experience of exclusion. The reason why a researcher might usefully ask about exclusion, as we analyse a person's dream, is not to penetrate the manifest content in order to reveal its hidden kernel: what really happened. As Zizek has pointed out, Freud, in his analysis of dreams, was not concerned with the latent dream-thoughts themselves, but rather with the question, 'Why were they transposed into the form of a dream?' (Zizek, 1989, p. 11). I cannot say how participants *really* experienced exclusion. However, asking about the experience of exclusion brings forth a number of productive ways of seeing the event.

Accounting for exclusion in the present

The issue of pupils changing or leaving institutions (for example, changing schools from primary to secondary, mainstream to special or being excluded from school) has received little attention. Concerns tend to be about the effect of the provision. The focus may be on what led to the exclusion or whether the pupil is happy in the new school and what will be the impact of the change/exclusion on their child's future, rather than how the change *itself* is managed and experienced.

However, in recent years there has been some research on the experience of transition, which can itself have an independent effect on performance. Ann Rushton's (1995) work on the transition from nursery to reception class indicated that the effects of sudden change to 'big school' can be traumatic and the shock can have long-lasting effects on performance. Feelings of loss of control occur when sudden change is effected in environment. All too often, after a decision has been made about the form of educational provision a child will receive, the move is made rapidly, with little preparation. Furthermore, the opportunity to use the change to address issues of separation, feelings of rejection, anger and loss tend not to be taken up.

It seems surprising that teachers, who are so attuned to issues of trauma and separation which the child might experience in the home (from the work of Bowlby, 1973; see also Barrett and Trevitt, 1991) have tended not to address these concerns within the educational context. There tends to be little consideration of the sudden severance of attachment figures such as friends, a special teacher or reassuring routines. By exploring the meanings of exclusion, rather than what leads to the exclusion, or what are the consequences of exclusion, this approach moves away from the mainstream psychological focus on developmental sequences (Burman, 1994a). In the interviews, I identify instances in which excluded pupils express anxieties, helplessness and responsibility for their plight, fears about staying in control and uncertainties about their future. Some employ educational and psychological discourses that seem to put the pain of rejection at a safe distance. This involves presenting extended quotations from several accounts to convey something of particular pupils' experiences. It is hoped that this approach will give a flavour of the multifarious and often conflicting nature of the accounts.

I discuss three interviews here with boys I call Ben, Charles and Philip. I also analyse the transcript of a discussion group, attended by six pupils, to discuss 'exclusion'. All the pupils were aged 12 or 13. Two of the pupils had been temporarily excluded. The school has high exclusion rates, with over 20 per cent of the pupils having been temporarily excluded at some stage in their school career. Finally, I interviewed the headteacher of the school.

The transcripts discussed here indicate that there was remarkable agreement among pupils about the consequences of exclusion. They catalogued a series of punishments from parents and carers, including confinement (they are 'grounded' and restricted in leisure activities), physical punishment and the imposition of a variety of chores. One difference in accounts seemed to lie in the way they spoke of the justification for exclusion. Some pupils' position themselves as having some responsibility for the exclusion. Their accounts are confessional and express a series of painful dilemmas about the event. Some pupils parodied the excluding authorities and reversed relations of power in their accounts of an exclusion taking place. Finally, some recounted the event in concrete terms, giving factual and abstracted information which was related to the topic of discussion. Each of these ways seemed to set up particular subject positions between myself as researcher and the interviewees. I end the discussion by speculating on the effects such styles of accounting had on my own experience of exclusion.

The interview as a site of resistance

A particular concern of this chapter is to explore the functions which the interviews and discussion had for the experience of exclusion. Did the interview regulate pupils or did the interview offer a site of resistance against deeper forms of governmentality? If we are to assess whether the interviews function to regulate or whether they succeed in offering a potentially transformatory space with which to deconstruct dominant constellations of power/knowledge, we must explore the effects which the excluded pupils' discourse has for the way they see themselves within the interview setting and its consequences.

It is helpful to pause for a moment to clarify what we mean by resistance. Within Newtonian physics, resistance is seen to operate by creating a barrier to the free flow of energy. If we apply the notion of resistance to the activity of excluded pupils, *vis-à-vis* her/ his interviewer or teacher, we are suggesting that s/he is blocking the activities of professionals. This might be done by undermining professional versions of the reasons for exclusion, or even the notion that there is a reason, which is located in a specific place (usually the head of the pupil).

Context of the research

It was recognized that the pupils' perception of me and where I stood in relation to school and social service authorities would require careful consideration. The context of the interview is also clearly particularly important. Pupils were interviewed during school time, by withdrawing them, either individually, or in groups, from their lessons. Such an approach had dangers of reinforcing the 'special' status of many pupils who have been excluded. The impact of talking to an outside 'visitor' (whether this is a researcher, educational psychologist or other 'professional') to the school should not be underestimated. It is possible that it could be experienced as being yet another humiliating ritual. The opposite risk, which seemed a greater concern for the teachers, was that the pupils would gain status among other pupils by being 'chosen' to help the 'lady'. While attempting to avoid being seen as either an 'ally' of the pupil, or a figure of authority, the tone of the interview was generally supportive. I tended to empathize most strongly with the excluded child. The following 'preamble' was given at the start of the interview.

> Hello. My name is Deborah. I am doing some research to find out what young people think about being excluded from school. I wonder if you'd be willing to help me by answering some of my questions, to help me understand what you think? . . . Before we start, I want to tell you that my work is not connected with [the school]. I am talking

to several young people from different schools and when I write about what they say, I will not use names or any details.

What pupils say about exclusion is clearly a response to the circumstances in which they are asked and how they make sense of our meeting.

Charles initially takes great care to provide me with a detailed account.

I: I just want to ask you some questions about how you felt generally about being excluded, so can I start off by asking you, is it, I know you've been excluded once. Have you been excluded any other times?

Charles: Which school? Which school? From this school?

I: Yes.

Charles: Erm, yes, I've been excluded a couple more times.

I: Right. When was that?

Charles: Er, I've been excluded . . . like, I've been excluded about two or three times before Christmas and er, I think it's once after Christmas, I've been excluded.

I: Right.

Charles: And er, I can't remember any others.

He struggles to cooperate with me and offers greater precision and detail than was requested. If we were to conceptualize the interview in terms of styles of gameshow, this would have resembled the format used on *Mastermind* (see Parker, 1989). Charles strove to produce the 'correct' answers. At the end of the interview, he seemed supportive of my efforts to find out about exclusion, and keen to reassure me:

I: Is there anything that you want to ask me, or tell me about being excluded, because maybe I'm not asking the right question. Really I want to understand what you think. Your point of view. Is there anything that would help me?

Charles: I can't think of anything. I think you're asking the right questions.

I: Thanks very much for coming. It's been really helpful. Um, okay. You've got a class now, haven't you?

After finishing the interview, when leaving the room, Charles said, 'Miss, will you be coming in next week? Can I come and speak to you again?' The interview thus seemed to be a mutually rewarding exchange. Charles seemed to have enjoyed the opportunity to air his grievances to an adult. He strove to offer an accurate account of his experience and feelings. The interviewer's role was to ask 'appropriate' questions and 'understand' what was being conveyed.

Other pupils welcomed the opportunity to make a more forceful protest, as in the following poignant extract:

I: And do you think it was fair that you were excluded?

Ben: I don't know, cos we were doing this lesson and everyone was making funny noises and blaming it on me, so when I was sent out of the room, this kid who I had a fight with, Matthew, he moved the chair that I was sitting on, and I fell over, so I just got mad at what he was doing. It made me really angry.

I: What did you do when you got angry?

Ben: I just hit out.

I: So what did you think when they told you you couldn't come to school?

Ben: [despairingly] It's not my fault. It's not my fault.

Charles' and Ben's interviews seemed to function in similar ways to a counselling session. They expressed strong feelings about their experience, as well as towards me as the person to whom they told their story. My sympathetic response of supporting protest seemed to open up some opportunity for pupils to resist their status as a 'problem' which needs to be removed. While a psychoanalytic interpretation would suggest that Ben has 'got in touch' with a sense of helplessness and despair, a Foucauldian interpretation (discussed below) suggests that the mirror held up to him in the interview draws him in to greater self-regulation – a more effective form of control than external regulation.

The interviews were markedly different from the tone of discussion of pupils who talked about exclusions in groups. They tended to adopt a much more playful attitude to the topic, conferring, debating and laughing at their own and others' foolishness. Using the gameshow analogy, the group interview took a less serious form, more akin to *The Price is Right*. There are no right or wrong answers. The main concern is how 'deliriously happy' participants are with their prize (Parker, 1989). They also tended to adopt a more teasing attitude towards me (accusing me of being a cockney, or laughing as I strove to work out what it was that I was missing). Thus the discussion groups formed an important site of pupil resistance to powerful adults, whether they were interviewers or teachers.

I: I want to start off by asking you, do you know anyone who has been excluded from school?

Sally: Yes.

Group: [Laughs.]

I: Does that mean you know someone or . . . ?

Jane: Well, I know one . . . [laughs]

Those in the group discussion tended to invert power relations and ridicule teachers. In the following discussion one girl talks of the circumstances surrounding her exclusion;

I: What did your parents think about it?

Sally: My dad just wanted to beat up Mr Thompson.

Group: [Laughs loudly.]

Sally: He don't even know how to run a [inaudible due to laughter] let alone a school. And he kept changing his story every time.

Power relations are reversed by the group. The teacher is exposed as being vulnerable to attack, ridiculous and a transparent liar. The interviews and discussions may have been the first time pupils had their views solicited by a 'grown-up' on the subject of authority structures, policy and practice in the school. While it has become a commonplace interviewing disempowered groups, to do so with pupils during school could rightly be construed as a subversive act.

Both the individual interviewees and the group challenged the legitimacy of excluding. But the group took this critique one step further by deconstructing the actions of teachers so that their arbitrary nature was exposed. Similarly, they transformed the role of researcher from someone who (potentially) knows, to one who is bewildered and lost. They demonstrated my ignorance of inside knowledge by excluding me from the joke. Relations of exclusion were thus overturned. In this way, the group assumed control by defining the flow of discussion.

Reflections on the ambivalent self

When talking about the fairness of being excluded Charles expressed ambivalent feelings. On the one hand, he complained that the teachers failed to recognize that he was not all bad:

Charles: She was telling them the bad side of me, she wasn't putting in any good parts at all.

I: Do you think it was fair that you were excluded permanently? . . . Is that the word you'd use to describe it?

Charles: It wasn't all that fair you know, in the last year, you know, it was only about a week in the last year there.

Deb Marks

I: A week to go?

Charles: No, no, er, that was . . .

I: Oh, you'd just begun.

Charles: Yes, just begun in the last year. I don't think it was fair in that way, you know, yes, other than that yes, cos like, I think that was from my behaviours.

Yet later on, Charles describes his punishment as having some justification.

I: So was that the worst part of being excluded?

Charles: Yes. So I had to make break up my punishment, but I think it was fair that . . . it's only fair, innit?

I: Is that what you think?

Charles: [smiles] Yes.

In conceding that his punishment may have been justified, Charles appears to become an 'agent' in his own self-regulation. He felt that one advantage of being excluded was that it could help him become 'conscious' of his behaviour.

I: So was that the best thing to do from their point of view, or do you think, did that help you in terms of . . .

Charles: It might have helped me a bit.

I: How would it help you?

Charles: Tell me like how I am in school you know, cos if I make mistakes, I'm just starting to get on with that you know, get on with that in school.

Ben exhibits similar conflicts over whether it was useful or useless and fair or unfair to exclude him, although generally he felt it was a wholly negative course to take. Early on in the interview I asked:

I: Did you feel that it helped, not coming into school for a few days?

Ben: Not really.

I: What happened when you were at home?

Ben: Nothing.

I: What did other people think about you being excluded?

Ben: Well, people in my class, some of them, me friends, said it wasn't me who started it. The kid that I told you about, he smacked me head off the table. So then . . .

But later on Ben (reluctantly) identifies some rational logic in the decision to exclude him. However, this logic does not indicate that he is in accord with the exclusion:

I: How do you feel about being excluded?

Ben: Some of the kids do bad things and they've got to be excluded. I do bad things and I did something bad so I had to be excluded.

Ben goes on to resist the assumptions behind his transitive inference, by suggesting other ways of dealing with the conflict he has with another boy:

I: Can you think of anything else [other than exclusion] that would help you?

Ben: Yes. If he [the boy Ben is in conflict with] changes rooms, classes.

I: It sounds like you have problems in that class. So you would like him to change.

Ben: He's my problem.

I: You seem sad about that. Has anyone asked you what you think the problem is?

Ben: No [inaudible, near to tears].

I: Is there anyone that you can talk to about what you think?

Ben [shakes head].

Ben went on to say that he was being teased and being called a 'tramp'. I tried (somewhat belatedly) to reverse my unthinking 'reflective' comments 'it sounds like you have problems . . . you seem sad' (used in counselling to encourage a client to 'stay with' her/his difficulties), since I realized that it would not be appropriate for Ben to get upset and then have to go back to class. But my attempts to move off the subject of his problems failed and a picture rapidly emerged of a child being bullied. Ben thus resists the interview format, although in doing so he engages in painful confession which increases his feelings of dependency. I seemed to be unable to withdraw from the position of rescuer:

I: You've been at the school for two years now. What do you like about the school generally?

Ben: One of the problems is that you come in and third years come up to you and ask you if you've got any money. They just keep coming up to you and ask you.

It thus became increasingly difficult to extricate myself from the role of 'counsellor', so we spent the rest of the interview looking at the strategies Ben might adopt to help the situation.

These accounts exhibit a number of conflicting feelings: of being under attack, feeling responsible, feeling guilty and innocent. Traditional quantitative research methods that strive to uncover underlying, unified 'attitudes' may well lose such complexity. Moreover, they fail to show the relationship between the interview context, the account and the positions offered to the various parties in the story.

Internal struggles and dilemmatic accounts

Many of the interviews can be characterized as describing 'internal' struggles. Charles, as with many interviewees, felt particularly insecure about whether he was capable of avoiding another exclusion:

I: So in terms of being excluded again, do you think that might happen?

Charles: Well, if I don't watch my way, yes. If I don't keep my mouth closed.

I: Do you think it's more likely to happen to you than anyone else?

Charles: Yes. I'm the worst, aren't I?

I: Are you? Would you agree with the way teachers see you? Would you see yourself in the same way, do you think?

Charles: Probably yes. The teachers know that I've got a good side to me as well, so I . . .

I: You've got?

Charles: A good side of me as well as a bad. So I . . . Yes.

Charles reflects on 'himself' and his different 'parts'. He must keep his mouth under control. He has a 'good' and 'bad' side, which are in a struggle for dominion. His account can be characterized as 'dilemmatic' (Billig *et al.*, 1988) if one is adopting a discursive approach, or 'ambivalent' if one is employing a psychodynamic discourse.

Ben felt similar anxiety about his ability to prevent another exclusion:

I: Do you think it will happen again?

Ben: I hope not. The kids still aggravate me, but I've learnt to control my temper.

A Foucauldian interpretation would suggest that Ben has become a self-governing, reflective citizen. Similarly, Charles reflects on forms of school discipline and the differing ways they support his attempts at self-regulation. He feels that the good side will prevail if he is closely monitored:

I: Yes . . . So generally you think that being excluded is reasonably fair in terms of what is happening at the time.

Charles: Yes.

I: That's what you would have chosen to happen.

Charles: Well, could have. But not as harsh, you know, like it's dead hard being excluded.

I: Yes. What would you choose as a punishment? Like what do you think would help you most, in terms of stopping you fighting and being naughty.

Charles: Er . . . I don't know. Like, now I'm on report. You get on report after being excluded. But most of the teachers find it better when I'm on report like, then I know someone is keeping an eye on me. So like, I'm always like, behaving more times than I usually am when I'm not on it, so they find it better when I'm on it. So like report, that would be a good idea. And like detentions and stuff like that, instead of always being excluded.

Not being able to predict their own behaviour or prevent the possibility of repeated exclusion seems to have left several pupils feeling insecure and vulnerable. In the above extract Charles counterpoises the harshness of exclusion with the positive effect of being on report. Yet he is speaking from the perspective of the teachers ('most of the time the teachers find it better'). Charles takes on the teachers' perspective as his own. Feeling that he is being monitored seems to be experienced as containing. Rose (1989) points out that the production and regulation of the normal child involves constant scrutiny. The pathological child is produced in relation to the production of the normal child. By contrast, the production of the pathological child seemed, in this instance, to involve the *absence* of scrutiny. Charles and Ben struggle to achieve a secure place within school, symbolized by bringing themselves under disciplinary gaze. Yet they describe the path of keeping their weaknesses and idiosyncrasies under control, such as the tendency to 'lose control' as one fraught with dangers and pitfalls. The regulatory discipline that brings Ben and

Charles into the view of authorities is experienced as more benign than exclusion, which renders them invisible.

Concrete disengagement versus abstract confession

While the above accounts of exclusion are replete with dilemmas about the experience of being excluded, some pupils gave accounts that were devoid of conflicts or anxieties. Philip's account is quite unemotional, to the point of removing any reference to himself from the account. He also seems to be uninvolved in the interview. Events and incidents are described concretely, as if they were being observed by an outsider rather than an involved party. The event is relayed systematically and without strong emotional expression:

> *I*: Basically, I want to ask you about exclusions because I think you've been excluded. Is that right?
>
> *Philip*: Twice.
>
> *I*: When were the times?
>
> *Philip*: Can't remember.
>
> *I*: Is it a while ago?
>
> *Philip*: Three months ago.
>
> *I*: Right. And can you remember how long it was for?
>
> *Philip*: Indefinite.
>
> *I*: And how long did that work out for?
>
> *Philip*: One or two weeks.
>
> *I*: Did they tell you, they didn't give you much idea what it would be that would decide that you could come back?
>
> *Philip*: No. It was something that I didn't do, I got excluded for it. They said I bullied Tom and stuck his head down the toilet.

Philip resists the attempt of the interviewer to adopt the position of a 'befriender' who wishes to 'hear his story'. His refusal to enter into a confessional discourse forces me into the position of asking concrete questions about facts. In resisting the disciplinary gaze of the researcher, he is removing himself from reflective involvement in the process of moving from being part of the school to being excluded from it. Philip avoids using personal pronouns. The situation exists outside himself. His account is laden with jargon that seems to distance him from involvement in the situation he is describing. Later on I asked:

I: What did you feel about the decision to exclude you the first time?

Philip: They did it indefinitely at first, and then sent a letter to say it was permanent.

I: Right, so you were just at home and then they said you couldn't come back. What happened when you were at home? What was that like?

Philip: I was off school for about four months.

I: It's quite a long time, isn't it?

Philip: Then I come to this one.

A question about experience is interpreted factually – in terms of what happened. Control was seen as being a purely external phenomenon. Dialogue with the self is absent in Philip's account. I occupied the position of forcibly extracting information. Philip's answers are only indirectly related to my questions, rendering the questions redundant. Despite my attempts to position myself as empathic ally, Philip resists the interview format and makes it clear that he is attending the interview under sufferance.

A professional account

The teacher interviewed tended to avoid discussion of their role and the role of the school in excluding. Responsibility often seemed posited with parents and, to a lesser extent, the child. When she was asked about the specific way a pupil would be told that they were to be excluded, the answer dealt with what is generally said to all pupils rather than how a specific incident might be managed:

I: I was wondering how you go about excluding. I mean, what is actually said and erm . . .

Teacher: Right, I mean, right, well what is said generally, I mean, it is something that we talk quite a lot about, especially when children come in to the school. We make it very clear that we don't like to have children out of school, because on the one hand we're saying you must attend, you must attend, and it does seem, the logic of it does seem barmy at times . . . we make it clear in assemblies and in tutorial session why people are excluded.

A step is taken away from the specific events surrounding exclusion and how it is accomplished, towards a general justification for exclusion. This has a distancing effect, keeping the painful event and how it is managed at bay.

The teacher argues that temporary exclusions (the interview took place before the 1993 Education Act outlawed this form of exclusion) are carried out in order to bring parents into school. She read out record cards of three pupils to me, who had been excluded for 'defiance':

> *Teacher*: What it actually says on this exclusion letter is defiance. Er, but he, as well as that, he's been um, bullying another child . . . And a third one, again, it's defiance, but again, based on a history of behaviour and a lack of parental involvement.

The vague category of defiance is interpreted as 'bullying', 'behaviour' and 'lack of parental involvement'. This latter rationale lays bare the way in which the pathologization of the pupil's parents plays a central part in the pathologization of the child (Donzelot, 1980). While categories for excluding pupils change over time, the teacher's account tends to be general rather than specific, placing pupils into fixed categories in the same way that social psychologists place their 'subjects' into fixed boxes. The teacher also posits the origins of the problems in external events which are wholly absent in pupils' accounts:

> *Teacher*: When something does erupt in the school, it's actually as a result of something that happens outside school . . . so it's things that go on outside that were actually brought into school.

In this way, the disorderly 'outside' may contaminate the rational rule-bound school. The image here is one of an explosion. 'Something erupts' and it becomes necessary to remove offenders and have a cooling-off period. Yet this image of a sudden event is moderated by the teacher's insistence that exclusion is mostly only resorted to after a long sequence of 'incidents'. The implication is that exclusions are disorderly events which can nevertheless be predicted by the monitoring activities of the school.

Conclusion

I have only briefly reviewed some of the different accounts of exclusion offered in discussion groups and individual interviews. The aim of the research has been to enrich our understanding of exclusion as a discursively constituted, institutionally bound and lived experience. The interviews showed something of the complexity of the thoughts and feelings of young people regarding exclusions. They rarely feel either all bad and culpable or totally free from responsibility. When asked about the reasons for exclusion, the answers given are quite specific. Most focused on the complex series of events around the exclusion, involving interactions with the school, teachers and parents. These factors are placed in an historical context and pupils often felt able to identify patterns which may lead to further exclusions. Some pupils gave accounts which positioned themselves in a variety of conflicted ways. Others resisted the normalizing moves of the 'dilemmatic' discourse and positioned themselves outside the struggles associated with exclusion. This latter rhetorical move seems to have more in common with professional accounts. In the interview with the head teacher of the school, an account of exclusion was offered which positioned the excluded pupil as being isolated from their social context.

When entering the world of exclusion, emotions associated with the event can be quite painfully re-experienced. Some pupils expressed conflicts and uncertainties about why it happened and where responsibility for the exclusion lay. This may be because the danger of repeated exclusion is ever-present. By contrast, other pupils seemed to have brought the event under control and turned it into 'facts'. This seemed to be achieved by disengaging from the experience of being excluded and by talking about it as if it were a neutral event rather than something in which they were involved.

This analysis of pupils' experiences of exclusion has employed a close textual analysis of the function that language has in the way pupils and teacher present themselves. The use of abstraction, confession and protest all represent different strategies for dealing with an important life event. However, I have not attempted to analyse the underlying motivation of the small group of people interviewed. Such an endeavour would be ontologically and methodologically suspect. I have also tried to avoid establishing an opposition between emotional, conflicted and hence 'authentic' accounts and generalized, jargon-laden 'inauthentic' accounts. Rather, the focus has been on the structure of the accounts and the way in which feelings and facts were produced in the context of the research setting.

This discussion has focused on the meanings of exclusion, rather than inclusion. As such, inclusion seems to function as an unmarked term, a normal, unquestioned state. This asymmetrical approach to the terms exclusion and inclusion seems to have been mirrored in the experience of carrying out the interviews. Where the interview felt collaborative, as in those discussions characterized by conflicted, ambivalent discourse, the interviewer was offered a self-affirming position as benevolent counsellor or researcher who had succeeded in establishing 'rapport'. By contrast, the disengaged discourse denied the interviewer a 'vantage point' into the 'soul' of the excluded subject. If one is to adopt a psychoanalytic perspective and use countertransferences as a research tool (Hunt, 1983), it is possible to speculate that the latter (disengaged) discourse offers the interviewer a more direct *experience* of the feelings of exclusion.

Deb Marks

Notes

1 An earlier version of this chapter was published in *Children and Society*, 9(3), 1995.
2 This research was funded by the Susan Isaacs Fellowship, Institute of Education, London University.

Part III

Dis/locating institutional boundaries

Psychological discourses are deployed in a wide range of locations in contemporary Western cultures. Like other chapters in this book, each of the following chapters focuses on a site at which psychology functions to define and regulate the achievement of 'normality' by the individual. The particular contribution of the chapters in this section is to challenge the idea that these discourses operate as all-powerful or totalizing. In this part we highlight the resistance to dominant discourses in the form of counter positions, or locations in which their implications are not as might have been predicted. Notwithstanding psychology's centrality in creating regimes of truth about ourselves (and our relationships with parents, children, lovers and friends), attending to specific contexts of performance enables the recognition of resistance as well as regulation.

Each of the chapters here illustrate how subject positions are mediated by institutional webs of discourse and how technologies of reading/inscription are constructed and perfomed. The institutional sites that are taken as topics are psychological expertise on parent–child relations (Chapter 8); the cultural representation of women in relation to humour (Chapter 9) and the gender reassignment clinic (Chapter 10). All these institutions are constructed and maintained through psychological discourses of gender and individuality, with boundaries drawn between and among categories of women, men, mothers, parents and children. Whether deployed by professionals or by others, psychological discourses produce powerful effects in these contexts through their practices and technologies of categorization. Technologies are understood here as occupying a range of positions as regards their materiality: from linguistic technologies of power that wield power through knowledge, to material technologies that exert their power by inscribing our bodies and our material existence.

The key regulative practices of these normalizing discourses are: in Chapter 8, the self-education of parents and the consequent self-regulation or government of their relationships with children – in advance of possible institutional interventions and assessments; in Chapter 9, the public absence of women's humour and the corresponding positions assigned women who use humour, as a transgression of passive femininity; and in Chapter 10, the control of access to gender reassignment programmes, including the exclusion of those who do not (or do not wish to) meet the conventional definitions of femininity and heterosexuality.

The focus of this part is on how government by psychological discourses does not only happen through our interpellation within them by professionals, since we also come to construct ourselves and the meanings of our experiences through these discourses. It is in this sense that such psychological discourses are productive. They form part of the culturally available meanings through which we produce ourselves as subjects. Thus while being intimately tied to certain institutional forms and practices, regulatory discourses are not confined to, nor wholly contained within, these. Rather, they operate across and beyond the disciplinary boundaries that are drawn up around us, such that they produce us in their image.

This part examines the ways these productive discourses act through the formation of the subject both to regulate and yet also to provide the means for resistance. We therefore highlight the tensions that emerge from a close analysis of the processes by which various positions may be adopted: by means of such de/constructionist readings we identify tensions, disagreements and impurities which provide potential strategies for resistance. These disagreements can be found in the apparently contradictory coexistence of environmental and maturational ideas in discourses of child development; in the regulatory but enabling features of humour and its links with desire and the politics of the unconscious; and in the many local and global technologies (including generative tensions, aetiological doubling and ambiguities of 'racial' and sexual identifications) of gender identity clinics.

Thus Chapter 8 highlights how a close scrutiny of psychological discourses allows us to see surprising coexistences in discourses of expertise of childrearing that challenge the apparently global and uniform discursive effects the discourse of psychological development is sometimes assumed to produce. In Chapter 9 the concept of 'carnival' is developed to see humour as a political strategy that can be transformative, rather than simply containing dissent as a form of 'repressive tolerance'. Finally, Chapter 10 draws on the notion of the boundary object to highlight both regulatory sexual policies and strategies of resistance performed across and between institutional boundaries and their technologies of inscription.

Chapter 8

Whose expertize?
Conceptualizing resistance to advice
about childrearing

Pam Alldred

Psychological discourses present themselves as authorities on our intimate relationships. Psychology's knowledge of 'the child' and 'his [sic] development' makes it the expertise *sine qua non* in the realm of parent–child relations and childcare practices in contemporary Western cultures.[1] Within this domain, as in others, psychological discourses can clearly be understood as regulative. This chapter illustrates the change in tone from the experts who advised mothers earlier this century, to the way psychological knowledge about children is presented to today's parents who are obliged to be informed by it. Does this shift reveal any change in the power of psychological discourses? Does a discursive framework (Foucault, 1977a, 1979, 1980a; Parker, 1992) allow us to recognize the power of psychological discourses of mothering without constructing women as passive in relation to them? How might we conceptualize women's active engagement with and resistance to psychological discourses of motherhood?

Currently in the UK, a popular forum in which advice on child-rearing is presented is in glossy parenting magazines. This is a relatively new forum for such material. The 'manuals' of mothercraft and infant care published throughout the past 50 years have attracted considerable attention from historians of child-rearing practices (Newson and Newson, 1974; Hardyment, 1983) and feminist critics for their normalizing and blaming of mothers (Marshall, 1991; Singer, 1992). Feminist commentators such as Ehrenreich and English (1979) have criticized the role of the (male) expert in relation to mothers. However, perhaps their analysis of the expert – which implicitly draws on a Marxist model of ideology and social control – is less appropriate in relation to contemporary parenting magazines. An examination of the way contemporary advice is presented will suggest that a more appropriate focus for examining its authority is on the 'discourse' itself. Second, their approach is limited as regards its provision for considering the role of desire in the production of subjectivity. Feminist understandings of power and resistance in the lives of women demand a more sophisticated analysis than simply of the weight of ideology. In the final section, I begin to explore how a discursive approach might avoid these pitfalls and how resistance to expert discourses on the child might be recognized in some of the everyday acts of individual subjects as well as in organized political resistance. First, some historical background on advice to mothers.

The expert advises mother

At the start of this century, in the West, the advice experts were giving to mothers focused on the physical health of infants. By the middle of the century, the psychologist had usurped the medical doctor as key expert on 'the child' (Ehrenreich and English, 1979; Hardyment, 1983). Outlining some of the changes in advice reveals something of how authority has been retained despite fairly rapid changes in the actual practices recommended. The content of rolling waves of advice will be significant for the discussion later of domains for its contestation.

For about the first 20 years of the twentieth century, an ethos of hygienism predominated and this persisted through the shift from physical to psychological care (Newson and Newson, 1974). Absolute regularity in feeding, sleeping and toileting and limited cuddling and holding characterized the advice of experts from the late 1920s into the 1930s (Urwin and Sharland, 1992). These abstemious qualities continued with the reign of experts such as J. B. Watson, who firmly warned against the dangers of 'mollycoddling' babies and creating weak, undisciplined, hedonistic individuals (Newson and Newson, 1974; Hardyment, 1983). Urwin and Sharland (1992) note the way the Second World War provided the context for an explicit regimentation of mothering and the imperialist motives for increasing attention to the development of the child.

The 1930s expert advice on the child is commonly characterized as environmentalist, with the predominance of ideas about how knowledge of the child's learning in response to environmental influences might be put to effective use in the production of better adjusted children. However, a different way of thinking about the child that emerged around this time is illustrated in the work of Arnold Gesell. His descriptions of developmental processes and maturation locates these actions and the 'stimulus' for them within the child. Although apparently logically opposed, these ideas did not shake 'the behaviourist stranglehold': instead 'developmental norms mapped neatly on to the prevailing morality which both endorsed self-sufficiency and yet also ensured considerable readiness to adapt to external demands. Indeed, in Gesell's scheme, accommodation was both normal and natural' (Urwin and Sharland, 1992, p. 183). 'Environmentalism' and 'developmentalism' were not necessarily operating as contradictorily at this time as one might expect.

After the Second World War, the general shift in emphasis changed the tasks of parenting from one of the control and management of the child's health and character to one in which surveillance and nurturance of the child's mind and emotions was emphasized (Rose, 1989). The influence of psychoanalytic thinking, particularly the work of Susan Isaacs, placed the emphasis on understanding the child's perspective; since the child's emotions might be reasonable, parents should try to understand them. Conceptualizing emotional development as something complex overtook the idea of emotions as simply fuelling progression along an already mapped route (see Urwin, 1985; Burman, 1994a) and this then allowed a discourse of individual differences to emerge which not only admitted both environmental and child-originating aspects, but constructed the child as an active subject in their world of relationships. Indeed, the complexity and relational nature of the child's emotional development was foundational for conceptualizing what is now the 'parent–child relationship' (Urwin and Sharland, 1992). Since this approach accorded the child aggressive as well as loving feelings it became possible for the child to be seen as in conflict with their environment. Newman, in 1914, had stated that 'the environment for a child is its mother' (c.f. Urwin and Sharland, 1992) and this is the starting point for D. W. Winnicott: mothers provide the environment for the infant and are thus responsible for their physical, emotional and psychological health. Recognizing the potential for conflict allowed the possibility that the interests of the child and of the mother might not be harmonious.

Today, it is not physical or spiritual, but psychological health that is the primary concern for most parents in the West. The relative luxury of a concern for psychological rather than physical health (Newson and Newson, 1974) for most, though sadly not all, Western parents does not somehow correspond to a lessened *degree* of concern for children. Instead, this opens up new areas of concern and raises new questions as to what adequate parents must be and do.

This brief historical account allows the identification of the traces of elements of different 'discourses' in advice literature today. Riley (1983) and Rose (1989) examine the conditions of possibility for these shifts, but the focus here is on the role of the expert. The term discourse is being used here to refer to a set of concepts and social practices through which we understand an object (Foucault, 1977a, 1979, 1981; Parker, 1992; see also chapter 1). If we take child development as the object of interest, psychology provides the dominant discourses through which we think about it in contemporary Western cultures. Among these discourses, that of the child as needing to be socialized can be distinguished from the discourse of the child as an organism whose development is progressively unfolding (Reese and Overton, 1970; Gergen, Gloger-Tippelt and Berkowitz, 1990). These discourses support more directed, or more 'child-centred' child-rearing and educational practices (Walkerdine, 1984) respectively. In turn, such practices construct the children who are the subjects/objects of them. Thus, concrete social practices and their material consequences are incorporated into this definition of discourse (after Foucault, 1977a, 1981). While the distinction outlined above allows the identification of different discourses of child development, there are clearly moments of complex interrelation between them (for example, in the 1930s when environmentalist and maturational discourses were not necessarily in conflict) and the meanings they give mothering must be considered in the specific historical moment.

Psychological discourses, mothers and feminist critiques

Feminists have found good reason to criticize psychological discourses of motherhood (Urwin, 1985; Phoenix, Woollett and Lloyd, 1991) and the construction of mothers through ideas about children (Walkerdine and Lucey, 1989; Burman, 1991a). By virtue of women's positions as primary carers for children, together with the narrow focus on the infant–parent dyad as the key influence on a child (Riley, 1983), psychology constructs mothers as objects of surveillance and regulation. Since the emergence of the concept of 'mother–child relationship', childcare advice has become less concerned with the problems of managing difficult children or difficult child-rearing tasks and more about the problems of in/adequate mothering (Urwin and Sharland, 1992). Problematizing mothering makes it the key site of scrutiny and blame and leads to psychology's provision of particularly polarized subject positions for mothers to occupy. Such positions permeate the cultural meanings of motherhood and also sustain institutional forms within social services and the law (which would, in fact, sound unreasonable to us if they did not draw on psychological concepts). However, psychology's role in these cultural meanings has not gone uncontested.

Critical psychologists highlight the power of psychology to describe the normal and natural and hence pathologize children who do not conform to psychological norms (see Chapter 3). Women who do not fit the dominant cultural subject positions for women risk being pathologized (as Chapters 6 and 9 examine). This operates around mothers when, in public debate, the mothering of women deemed 'too young', 'too old', or whose relationships and/or sexuality do not conform to conservative images of mothers is presumed to be lacking (Alldred, 1995). In the realm of mothering, psychology replicates and reinforces particular cultural ideas about individuality, rationality and maturity. Through their association with children, discourses of nature abound and, fuelled by our emotional investments in children and our own fears of vulnerability (Burman, 1994b), the toleration of children or mothers/parents who are different from the norm is limited so that they rapidly become pathologized (O'Hagan and Dillenburger, 1995).

Burman (1994a) identifies how the assumption of a causal relationship between mothering behaviour and outcomes in terms of qualities of the child – the 'developmental myth' – justifies close scrutiny of mothers to ensure that 'our' children are to develop healthily. A model of education as 'investment' relies on (and reproduces) the 'developmental myth' and places increasing pressure on parents to stimulate their child in order that they capitalize on their potential.

The social 'ownership' of children, which is illustrated in discourses of concern for 'our children', is soon 'forgotten' when it comes to allocating blame for having raised 'bad kids'. Similarly, responsibility is rapidly re-individualized when questions about financial obligations are raised. It seems that the individualism and the narrow focus of psychology on a very limited sphere of influence on the child (which at most extends from the mother–infant dyad to include the household unit) works most perniciously when deployed to account for the negative influence on children.

Critiques of the role of the expert

Feminist and Marxist critics have described how the expert wields authority and fulfils a regulative, normalizing function (see Chapter 3) as a result of the status that is accorded them and expert discourse relative to alternative discourses. Writers such as Ehrenreich and English (1979) have described the rise of the expert in relation to the care of the infant and small child as a form of colonization by the male scientific expert of what, until then, had been an area of women's knowledge. Infant care was one of a series of spheres of knowledge (which had included healing and midwifery) that science, by virtue of its claims to a superior means of knowing, supplanted. Male attention might have provided recognition of the fact that raising children is indeed 'tricky business' and elevated mothers from the status of automatons of nature to which they were sometimes relegated. The 'rise of the experts' depended on the elaboration of a scientific approach to child-rearing. Science was presented as, above all, objective and impartial, yet it expressed all the racist, colonialist and masculinist assumptions of Western thought. The legitimation of men's interest in children (though initially only the white, class-privileged men who were deemed fit to represent the civilizing rationality of science) might have held hopes of broader social responsibility for child-rearing, but these hopes were not met. Instead, the male child-raising experts of 1950s Anglo–American cultures 'had no material help to offer, but only a stream of advice, warnings, instructions to be consumed by each woman in her isolation' (Ehrenreich and English, 1979, p. 184). Knowledge of raising children came to rely more and more on the studies of scientific experts and less and less on the experience of mothers, until mothers came to be seen not only as the major agents of child development but also as the main obstacles to it (*ibid*, p.185). This professionalization of the tasks of motherhood, rather than raising the status of mothers, constructed them as inadequate, ignorant or pathological (and their mothering potentially insensitive, neglectful or overbearing), in opposition to knowledgeable, objective and benevolent experts.

Psychological discourses on the child do not necessarily present new knowledge, but what is significant is the epistemological backing that ideas have once encased in the rhetoric of psychology because of its authority as expert and scientific knowledge. Problematizing psychological knowledge, in an account such as this, is not simply to condemn it as 'bad' knowledge (inaccurate or maliciously motivated), but to question the extent to which its authoritative status makes it so difficult to contest. It renders other forms (such as mothers' own knowledge) pathological or simply irrelevant. As Foucault (1980b) noted, the effect is such that alternative discourses are often not only depicted as inaccurate, but those espousing it are depicted as charlatans.

Childcare advice 'baby books' which contain sustained advice from one expert, with consistent style and format are still published (for instance, Stoppard, 1995). Rather than advising, they may be descriptive and chart how the child will be (or ought to be) growing and developing month by month. Burman notes that 'normative descriptions provided by developmental psychology slip into naturalised prescriptions' (1994a, p. 4), so that even a descriptive text functions powerfully to produce culturally specific sets of requirements of parents. In taking up the tone and manner that signify 'expert', the author of such texts can sound rather patronizing. Do today's parenting magazines adopt the same patronizing tone and what role is the expert attributed within them?

Parenting magazines

Parenting magazines are 'special interest' magazines about babies and children that address (variably) parents or mothers. Sometimes, even an explicit address to 'parents' is contradicted by the more frequent address and orientation of its articles to mothers. *Parents* is the title of a current-selling UK magazine which nevertheless genders its reader through references to 'your breasts' or 'your [post pregnancy] body' and articles such as 'Distant Dads' in which women write about what it's like when 'your partner' is never there when you need 'him'.[2] These monthly magazines are relatively cheap and widely available (although the fact that they have to be purchased – rather than being freely distributed as is healthcare literature on motherhood – brings questions of 'choice' to the fore as well as the consumption of products through advertising). Their colourful, magazine-style format makes them very accessible and appealing and more like popular monthly women's magazines than child-rearing books and manuals. Compared with child-development texts they have a broader remit and in line with this they do not take a consistent advice-to-parents format. They are a popular medium through which messages about what is viewed culturally as contemporary good childcare and parenting behaviour are communicated and particular consumer 'needs' are constructed (Burman, 1994a). Each issue contains a variety of formats and corresponding tones. The key form through which information on child health and development is provided are 1–4 page features, focusing on a different topic in each issue. Experts are consulted on issues within their certified field, sometimes in small caption-like comments and in response to readers' queries. A second form in which 'sharing experience' is a more explicit theme and yet which also acts to inform parents and promote particular constructions of child psychology, the role of parents and the concerns of good parents, is where a mother gives her account of her experiences. The overriding tone is of *support for* parents – from other parents, the magazine staff and experts. The 'invitation' to parents to think of themselves, their tasks and their relationships through the discourse of psychology echoes the way 'self-help' discourses encourage people to form themselves through, and thus regulate themselves within the terms of psychological or psychiatric thinking (as Chapter 2 examines).

The title of the 'letters page' to which parents write with queries in *Parents*, is 'Can We Help?' Whatever your problem, big or small, write to us and one of our experts will be able to help you.' The team of experts called on to answer questions marks a difference from the practice of the help pages of earlier women's magazines in which the page would be identified as belonging to, and all letters would be answered by, one figure, an 'agony aunt' whose wisdom was supposedly reflected in the fact that she (for example, Virginia Ironside, Clare Raynor, (Dr) Miriam Stoppard) was a 'household name'. In contrast, responses are from a panel of several figures, of specific and declared expertise. In July 1992, for example, this included midwives, breastfeeding counsellors, a clinical child psychologist, a 'nutritionalist and mother', and a Professor of Obstetrics and Gynaecology. Instead of appeals to their personality and general wisdom, it is their specific disciplinary expertise that is significant.

Mother and Baby magazine illustrates the tone of neutrality that accompanies what is, apparently, simply 'information', perhaps 'new' or 'better' information. It is sometimes superficially framed in a 'new way' as if it might otherwise insult readers by implying it is knowledge they do not already have. This facesaving reinforces the implicit moral imperative to be up-to-date with expert thinking. An empowerment discourse is often implicit in the way information is provided and practices suggested and sometimes there is an explicit 'it's up to you to decide'.[3] Today's experts wouldn't dream of telling parents how to raise their child: they simply 'help' them to make (the right) decisions. It is interesting to consider this presentation style as illustrating the commodification of knowledge: which line of expertise will readers buy? However, the powerful claim to science of psychological discourses and the many institutionalizations of psychological ideas would suggest that competing expertises (such as medicine, spiritualism or religion) might not operate in the 'free market' that this rhetoric assumes.

The reassurances to parents that 'you know best' and 'you know more than you think you do' were popularized by Benjamin Spock in the 1950s and 1960s (Parmenter, 1994) and is sometimes echoed faintly as a reassurance. It is tempting to imagine that experts mean this to be encouraging and confidence-inspiring for parents, not necessarily because they really believe that parents will naturally know what's best, but because, above all, 'studies show' that a 'happy mother makes for a healthy child'.[4]

The psychological discourses on parent–child relationships are not specific to this medium; a whole 'family' of professionals surround the family (Rose, 1989) and midwives, health visitors, GPs and pharmacists are authoritative sources of help and advice to mothers. However, they illustrate a broader shift from explicitly prescriptive advice and an authoritative tone to a more equal and empathetic tone where the emphasis is more often on supporting parents and, while informing them, helping them to gather knowledge and letting them decide how to act on the basis of this knowledge. The superior and patronizing authorial tone is replaced by a identificatory and confessional stance that belies any hierarchical relationship between reader and author, but invokes 'an expert' in specific ways and places.

From advice to knowledge

The tone of parenting magazines suggests a concern to appear knowledgeable and confident in their assertions and the process of sounding often leads them to generalize. The balance to be struck is between being perceived as well-informed and 'expert', yet not being too authoritarian or condescending. Experts are often introduced by the regular writers who staff the magazine, who, for example, title and introduce an article, then hand over to the expert after having announced their credentials to the reader. Alternatively, in confessional or mock-intimate style they raise 'their own' questions and concerns. Perhaps this helps to retain this construction of the relationship between magazine staff and readers as one of equals with the staff simply using their access to the experts for the wider benefit of parents. Both *Mother and Baby* and *Parents* present their staff as 'just like you'. The small photographs of staff are accompanied by identificatory descriptions such as that the consumer writer is the mother of an 8-year-old boy and 2-year-old twins, or that the fiction editor's daughter has just started high school, as opposed to writing or research credentials. This prompts an identificatory rather than hierarchical relationship with them, according them respect not because they 'are experts', but for their knowledge. Hence it is *expertise*, as opposed to *the expert*, which is the site of authority or holder of power.

This alignment of magazine staff with parents – that is, as parents who are interested in the same information/advice – might offer potential alignments *against* experts or against offending companies or organizations, without explicit commitment to such positions. The removal of a single authority and the range of formats for 'information' presents an evident multiplicity of expertise. This inevitably produces contradictions, although these are rarely acknowledged.

Over the last 40 years the shift has been from scientific advice *to mothers* to psychological knowledge *for parents*. This is correspondingly reflected in the ways psychological ideas have come to dominate how we speak of children: a shift from an advising to an informing role for experts and sometimes a changed orientation to parents rather than mothers. The key point here is that the transition to a consumer-driven role of expert knowledge places parents as consumers. As such it produces for them the moral imperative to seek out and assimilate the knowledges that will enable them to do their task well. This provides the market for monthly 'throw-away magazines', as opposed to books that might have been handed down from mother to daughter.

Since we already understand 'what children are' through psychological ideas and theories, we thus already presume that the most important tasks of parenting are psychological and vast areas of questions become possible about how best to parent a child well, without damaging them psychologically. Parmenter (1994) observed that by the 1970s mothers were going to their doctor not for advice, but for reassurance that what they were already doing was alright. Thus, mothering practices were already informed by expert discourses. The centrality of the expert is eschewed by Dr Spock but, as Urwin and Sharland (1992) note, this displaced rather than altogether removed 'him'.

Being up-to-date with current thinking on child psychology, being knowledgeable about 'the child' (or this particular form of knowledge of the child) is part of being a good 'modern' parent. Moral attributions attach to the effort one makes in order to keep oneself informed. The tone of advice has changed now that ordinary parents are expected to be able to draw on psychological discourses. Convinced of the value of psychology, parents need only have new concepts or findings presented to them without their translation into implications for practice. The expert doesn't perform in the way that he used to. Is his authority more fragile now because of greater competition from a range of expert discourses? Do parenting magazines indicate anything of a shift in the authority of the expert or of the psychological discourses around mothering?

Are the experts less powerful today?

Understandings of children and parenting are suffused with psychological meanings and indeed would not make sense to us today if they were not. However, while there may be a dominant framework within which questions about children and parents are formulated, there is no consensus. Instead the discipline holds differing versions of knowledge, or different discourses. While the tone of the expert may be less didactic and different expertises, or within them different discourses, may compete with each other, psychological concepts and theories do not appear any less authoritative. Epistemological challenges or straightforward rivalries that competing expertises present prevent there from being a single overall source of authority on child-rearing. However, the naturalizing of psychology's place in our explanatory frameworks, so that the relevance and authority of the discourse goes unquestioned, makes the discourse more powerful.

Psychology remains powerful with networks of institutions supporting it and supported by it. Ehrenreich and English (1979) provide a powerful critique of the role of experts in relation to women and some of the consequences of this for women, but their account risks conflating the historical authority of the male expert with the seemingly (non-gender-specific) authority of professional discourses on children. Obviously the model of an authoritative, patronizing male expert making prescriptions about how mothers care for their children cannot account for the mode through which all expert knowledge operates today. It is not wholly appropriate now that many child-related professions such as health visitors are staffed predominantly by women rather than men. Indeed, perhaps today other factors such as class, economic and educational differences, more frequently structure the power relationships between childcare professionals and mothers (Walkerdine and Lucey, 1989). What remains significant is the power of professional discourse to define. Thus, the powerfulness of a discourse of expertise needs to be separated from the power of the male expert and, indeed, any embodied expert.

Examining the power of the expert

Seeing the expert as exercising power over mothers retains the common liberal model of power as an entity that can be possessed and is applied 'top down' in a negative, inhibitory manner (Van Krieken, 1991). It produces the impression of advice as coercive, instructing mothers with the threat of sanctions if they do not obey. Of course sanctions do exist: the interventions of professionals, including in specific locations the law, are real enough, but to understand parents as avoiding behaviours that are defined as warranting these interventions in order to avoid legal sanctions is to misunderstand the nature of power in these discourses.

Powerful though psychological advice on child-rearing is, it does not operate simply coercively. It is not out of fear of reprisal that parents implement advice, but for fear of the psychological and moral consequences constructed *within* the discourse. If power did operate in this unidirectional way, it would be far less stable since it would be operating against our wills (Van Krieken, 1991; Rose, 1989). As Parmenter (1994) notes, being overtly patronizing or prescriptive to mothers simply would not work.

The limits of power

Women have not simply always obeyed expert advice. For some women implementing the advice has not been possible even given their wish to do so. For example, Watson's firm warnings to mothers of the early 1950s not to cuddle their babies too much for fear of 'mollycoddling' them could not simply be heeded by some working-class poor mothers who would hold their babies close to them in order to keep them warm in winter (Newson and Newson, 1974). However, even acknowledging that mothers have not always taken expert advice merely provides only two positions for them to occupy; as either accepting or rejecting the advice. Mothers are therefore characterized as grateful and obedient or, if they disregard the advice, as stubborn, malicious or abnormal.

In some Marxist critiques of ideologies of motherhood (e.g. Barrett and McIntosh, 1982) as well as in some radical feminist critiques of the institution of motherhood (e.g. Firestone, 1970) women can be understood as occupying one of only two subject positions: mother (collusive) or non-mother (resistive). A woman is either 'duped' by the rosy images of motherhood or has 'seen through' its ideological effects, in which case her 'realistic' perspective allows her to resist. This produces only outright rejection of mothering as anything other than passive. This simplifies the means by which women resist either the presumption of, or specific meanings attached to, motherhood.

Applying Ehrenreich and English's analysis of the childcare expert's advice would similarly produce a mother as simply either obedient or disobedient of the advice. In either case, the subject is treated as passive in relation to a powerful discourse, having only preformed options available. This either/or possibility retains the assumptions of a unitary subject who is invested in only one or other position and it therefore restricts a more complex exploration of how forces operate at a subjective level. To continue the earlier example; that Watson's regime was felt to be cruel and that women were torn between their desire to do what was advocated as the best thing (leave the child to 'cry it out') and their desire to comfort the infant, demonstrates that, subjectively, responses to advice may be complex and multilayered. In order to recognize (and stimulate) women's struggles with dominant psychological meanings of motherhood, it is important that we can acknowledge both the power of the discourse and the possibility of resistance to it.

Knowledge as productive

The regulative power of psychological discourses of mother and child is enforced through the positions of *other* (unnatural, pathological) mothers and of *other* (negative, deviant) outcomes of their mothering. But this repressive side of its power is not the whole picture. Foucault's later work around 'technologies of the self' emphasizes the productive, as opposed to simply repressive, nature of these powerful discourses and, furthermore, how they operate through our formation of ourselves as subjects (Martin, Gutmen and Hutton, 1988). Psychological discourses are then understood to produce what they describe. This productivity provides for the experiences and relationships which we find positive (e.g. the pleasure of feeling that we are witnessing a child's own development) and the positions from which we might resist dominant meanings as well as dominant meanings themselves (Foucault, 1979).

Discourses of child psychology are appealing because they promise us knowledge of a better way to relate to children. The onus on parents to ensure they are well-informed is acted upon not because the subject position of the ignorant, old-fashioned parent is (negatively) morally laden, nor through the coercive power of psychology. Our desire to do the best for children is genuine. To say it is produced through discourse is not to imply it is a 'false consciousness'.

The 'will to knowledge' of best care of the child illustrates what is meant by a disciplinary (as opposed to a disciplined) society (Miller, 1987). Its effects are not only confined to the overt subjects of its institutionalized practices. Rather, all of us feel these effects even as we consciously take a critical perspective towards such practice. Not 'obeying' expert advice is not to escape its influence. Parents who reject the accepted best practice are susceptible to guilt and self-doubt. They are constructed as self-indulgent and potentially to blame for their children's inadequacies. The obeyed/disobeyed polarity posits the conflict somehow 'outside' the individual, whereas positing advice as powerful in our formation means it is formative of, rather than in opposition to, our will. We have come to understand ourselves, our experiences and relationships through psychological discourses (Gergen, 1989; Rose 1989); as contemporary Western subjects we are formed through the 'psy-complex' (Ingleby, 1985; Rose, 1985).

Given this productivity of discourse, is psychology all-powerful? Feminist writers who find Foucauldian analytics of power useful describe how even dominant discourses (such as psychological ones in relation to parent–child relationships) are powerful, but are not in possession of total power (Weedon, 1987; Sawicki, 1991; Bell, 1993). Such discourses are not closed systems of meaning, but remain contested and contestable through challenges at the micro-level. This might then meet the requirement for a framework that can recognize both how difficult are some options that are made and yet how some people still take them up: that is, an analysis of the power of a discourse, which does not imply it is a totalizing monolithic structure. Does a Foucauldian approach (Rose, 1989; Foucault, 1980b; Van Krieken, 1991) in which resistance, like power, is ever-present, offer a useful analytics, or does the assertion that 'resistance is everywhere' reduce organized resistance to the status of something haphazard and inevitable?

Resistance at the level of identity: to be, or not to be, a mother

Kaplan states that the 'given' of motherhood for women has been irrevocably called into question (Kaplan, 1992). Although she writes from a North American vantage point, several recent articles in British women's magazines would suggest a similar pattern for the UK ('The mother of all decisions: not everyone should have a child', *Cosmopolitan*, July 1994; 'Choosing no children', *Everywoman*, November 1993; 'Having a baby?', *She*, March 1994). It would seem that the sound-images 'woman' and 'mother' are not as conflated as they were in the past; that 'things are now more complex' (Kaplan, 1992). Direct and indirect pressures still exist, but resisting them and resisting the pathologization of non-motherhood is likely to be easier than it was for previous generations of women for, while impacting differentially on women, there may be a greater range of alternative 'identities' available. Other aspects of identity (such as those provided by/in the sphere of employment) may provide some women with discursive positions from which to resist the cultural pressure to procreate and find positive alternative identities. With (some) control over conception for heterosexual women and the (technical) possibility of entering the workforce, many more questions about identity open up for women today than in the past. Whether or not to have a child is one of them. If one aspect of this relates to a weakening of the association of woman with nature, perhaps it is a result of challenges to the discourse of 'the natural' made by organized resistance through feminist, gay liberation and 'queer' movements.

Marginal mothers

Women who choose to mother without men, such as those who are lesbians or never-married, single heterosexual women, can be understood as challenging the dominant assumptions that mothers must be in heterosexual relationships and that family – if that is what we call the intimate relations of care surrounding children – must be the 'nuclear family'. In this sense, lesbian mothers can be seen as challenging both the association between heterosexuality and motherhood and the construction of lesbians as disinterested in or hostile to children, or as psychologically unfit to mother (see Alldred, 1995). They may also challenge some of the homogenizing assumptions sometimes produced within lesbian and gay cultures (Lewin, 1994). Perhaps the 'lesbian baby boom' – the increasing numbers of lesbian mothers (or their increasing recognition) – is one element that prises apart the association of motherhood with naturalness and of unnaturalness with lesbianism.

Lewin locates the resistive feature of lesbian mothers in their existence. Certainly, they testify to the fact that, despite intense cultural pressures around (hetero)sexuality and motherhood, some individuals still occupy oppositional spaces, serving as a reminder that the hegemonic discourses are not seamlessly all-powerful (Weedon, 1987; Sawicki, 1991). However, this raises questions about how broadly we wish to define resistance. Are the everyday lives of mothers who did not choose their position as *other* in relation to 'normal motherhood' to be understood as resistance? Are the identities and psychic formations necessary for some people's self-preservation to be understood as political resistance? Do we want to distinguish between conscious acts of resistance and the very existence of mothers who are forcefully constructed as deviant, unfit or marginal? Does this distinction always hold? Might a discursive understanding of resistance transcend distinctions between volitional and non-deliberate acts, as well as between conscious and unconscious resistance?

Resistance at the level of identifications within discourse

While recognizing these 'global identity' options as potential resources for resistance, they do not represent the whole means by which women relate to the dominant discourses of motherhood, for this would leave the inadequate 'either/or' of subject positions described above. Discursive approaches direct analytic attention to more precise sites of resistance than individual 'identity' (Parker, 1992; Butler, 1993b; Mills, 1994). Deconstructing the model of the subject assumed within identity categories shows how it occludes the complex, shifting and, at times, contradictory ways the meanings of these identities operate. Critiques of the concept of identity have been developed through approaches associated with post-structuralist ideas in the fields of sociology, literary criticism, communication and media studies. These demonstrate that the representation of a person through the concept of identity presumes stability, fixity and internal coherence on the part of the individual and that, in actuality, lack of closure around identity means that neither one, nor a string of terms, exhausts the possibilities for describing a person. In order to explore the power of a discourse, it is necessary to examine the minutiae of how contestations of it are lived at the level of the manoeuvres an individual might make (Walkerdine and Lucey, 1989).

To speak of multiple identities available for women is not to imply that no practical constraints operate. An identity as mother can probably not be 'thrown off' for more than a limited time period; however, a mother may be able to negotiate certain of its meanings and mobilize other aspects of her identity to key significance at particular times. There will be times when, for instance, being a lesbian is significant and is operating against a woman's identity as a mother and times when this does not operate as a contradiction. There may also be times when, despite being cast as a contradiction, the actual meanings of the identities and the contradiction are different: for example, in heterosexual or gay defined contexts.

At the level of the individual, manoeuvres between different subject positions occur even when reading a text through which multiple subject positions operate. Approaches to film theory, communication studies, etc. have developed around concepts such as (multiple) identifications rather than (unitary) identities in order to produce this degree of flexibility and shifting subject positions rather than fixed readings that are guaranteed by the reader's identity.

Parent/mother

Women may be able to renegotiate aspects of the relations between themselves, their children and their children's fathers by taking up the subject
position of 'parent' as opposed to 'mother' and hence resist some of the
meanings that accompany 'mother'. However, the increasingly common practice in the UK of referring in public discourse to 'parents' rather than 'mothers' cannot be met with any simple, unitary evaluation. While many welcome
the way it shifts the onus of responsibility for children from mothers on to
mothers and fathers, it is unwelcome where it functions to obscure either the
actuality (that most 'parenting' work is still done by mothers) or the real
differences of power that exist between men and women. Like the gender
neutral terms elsewhere (e.g. Smart, 1989), mothers are disadvantaged by the
assumption of initial equity between mothers and fathers. The political implications of this discursive shift for mothers (or indeed for any particular
mother) are not simple or predictable. They can be positive or negative in
different locations. Switching between discursive subject positions of mother
and parent may sometimes be of little significance to a mother, yet may at
other times be mobilized in order to contest their elision.

Resisting expert discourses

Radical Motherhood and *Mothers Know Best* are particular examples of organized, or explicitly politicized, resistance. They are independent publications 'by parents, for parents' which take a critical stance to the advice of the
experts. Such forums are important sites of resistance. This section will briefly
outline how the strategies employed in *Radical Motherhood*, when understood
through a discursive framework, can be seen to exemplify the discursive manoeuvres that individuals too may make in reading parenting literature. The
voluntary nature of this publication and its refusal of commercial support
makes it an insecure location, but it serves to illustrate the forms of resistance
that are to be found more generally.

    Radical Motherhood is a north-east London-based monthly subscription
magazine that is broadly informed by feminist, critical and anti-consumerist
political perspectives. It has a different relation to consumer products than the
'glossies', both because it does not take advertisements and because of its
articulated anti-consumption theme. It produces a more explicit alignment
between readers and writers. The spaces into which readers are welcomed are
significantly different. Parents are encouraged to write articles, to comment on
and disagree with particular articles or the magazine overall. The writers
appeal for other local parents to contribute and to influence the direction
taken by the magazine. This is different from the ways parenting magazines
invite contributions which are circumscribed by the formats of the particular

sections, for example in sections called 'Say Hello! Here's your chance to air your views', 'Mums in Touch (Make a friendly pen pal)' and in problem pages and columns where an expert's advice is sought and consumer questions are answered. There are no pre-set forums or styles for readers' contributions and journalistic pieces are welcomed.

A key theme is the critique of professional intervention around childcare, health and childbirth and a 'know your rights' approach is taken at times. Some of the articles deploy detailed, radical arguments on specific issues, such as critiques of allopathic (mainstream) medicine relating to debates about the innoculation of children. Its small circulation is probably mainly among parents who are politicized and highly educated with relative independence from, and confidence in the face of, professionals. It exhibits a combination of strategies including undermining the warrant of expert discourses and asserting the right to be autonomous and self-directed in one's child-rearing.

Competing discourses

It is from the plethora of the circulating motherhood discourses that women take up subject positions. Without implying that they are equally available to different women or all equally persuasive, they can be understood as providing possibilities for making alternative meanings. Kaplan notes the historical continuities within the contemporary repertoire and how contemporary representations 'appear to gather up all of the past images as well as introducing new ones' (1992, p. 181). Therefore theories that are discredited or out of vogue may still be part of the cultural repertoire and so provide alternatives.

Contradictions provided within the magazines, for example, on different pages of the same issue, or between advertisers' messages and experts' advice, are even unsurprising given the fractured nature of the magazine contents. For mixed media such as magazines, semiotic analyses like that of Wicomb (1994) can be useful for studying discourses of motherhood and the way individual readers may make sense of these discourses. Contradictions between the meanings of statements and images provide possibilities for alternative readings.

Discursive positions need not be directly contradictory in order to provide positions of resistance against each other; they may operate within different registers. For instance, where medical and psychological discourses are in competition, it might be possible for psychological discourses to attain authority by implying a moral superiority of concern for the emotional needs of the child over what can then be constructed as a limited biologically mechanistic discourse of medicine. It could be presented as a more sophisticated concern (as opposed to a basic concern with physical health), or a newer way of seeing or doing things.

The child and good childcare practice is an example of the particularly rich repertoire containing discourses of very different types, including folk psychology, 'old wives' tales' and commonsense as well as rolling layers of expert knowledge forms. Within the same discipline, drawing on a different discourse of the child constructs a different role for mother or parent: alternative discourses of the child which emphasize either their self-regulatory or their impressionable qualities produce different degrees of responsibility or blame for parents. The discourse of the child as acutely impressionable and vulnerable to influences implies that environmental factors (of which parental influence is often the only one considered) are of greatest significance. In order to resist the parent-blaming consequences that this discourse can have, a discourse of the child as an unfolding organism with self-regulatory qualities could be drawn on. Such a discursive shift could enable a mother to resist being blamed wholly for her child's behaviour or character. Another option might be to insist that, within an environmentalist discourse, the parameters of influence are extended beyond the usual family/household (or even mother–child dyad) in order to acknowledge the role of the wider cultural influences on a child. More abstractly, the cause-and-effect links of the developmental myth can itself be criticized.

Contesting expertise: 'mothers' knowledge'

Another strategy is to undermine the status of the discourse one wants to resist. A mother's own knowledge gained through experience of mothering might be understood as what Foucault called a subjugated knowledge: one accorded lower status than scientific knowledge. However, that it is subjugated but not silenced is illustrated by the way it does exist as an alternative. Gergen (1989) describes different ways of warranting a preferred discourse. One way is to make an explicit reference to the source of the discourse or to how that knowledge is known. A mother can draw on a discourse of experience to support her knowledge in opposition to psychological knowledge. By explicitly claiming that her means of knowing is through experience, there can be an implicit (or explicit) criticism of the psychological discourse – which is constructed, by contrast, as abstract and ungrounded in practice. Her experiential knowledge might be grounded, for instance, in her knowledge of her particular child, or of their previous encounters with this issue, or of her experience with her other child. It may invoke the knowledge of her own mother. In the same way a phrase like 'Well, that's the *theory*, anyway' counterposes theory with practice where talk (theory) is easy but practice is what counts. This can be understood as an implicit epistemological challenge; a challenge to the means by which psychological discourses are warranted.

Critics of developmental psychology have shown the abstract, universalizing tendencies produced by the idea that 'the child' is an entity and hence knowable. These are challengeable by a mother's own claim to experiential knowledge of particular children, in particular circumstances. This can be bolstered by either humanist discourses of individual uniqueness or of theoretical critique of universalizing claims.

Changes in advice: 'taking it with a pinch of salt'

This example illustrates a general point about how change in advice occurs. Rather than being disproven in any unequivocal way, more often other discourses merely supersede it. They may differ in emphasis or may be about a different quality that is identified. But either way, that superiority tends to be assumed without rational or explicit contestation. Because neither the expert nor the discipline are univocal, advice cannot change instantaneously in any complete way, leaving possibilities for alternative formulations on a specific issue.

Mothers who experience dramatic changes in the advice they received for their second child compared with their first may elaborate through this position of resistance to advice *per se*, or to particular advice – either because they can point out its changing nature or because they can draw on previous specific alternative advice. Hardyment (1983) notes the role of commentaries (including her own) in demonstrating how historical changes in advice to mothers have even made dramatic turnarounds in the space of a few years. Showing historical or cultural variability undermines the claims science makes to universal knowledge.

Discourses or the subject positions within them are not necessarily identifiable as resources for regulation or resistance in general terms. This must not mean, however, that we are blocked from identifying damaging and oppressive relations, but that they might be more usefully conceptualized in terms of specific subject positions and locations. For instance, identifying a moment at which, for a particular woman, the idea that she constitutes the child's environment in its entirety has oppressive consequences avoids the overgeneralization that every potential subject position around motherhood is 'bad for women'. Such specific assessments are called for in order to take account of the way a discourse is functioning in a precise cultural context. Instead of either/or subject positions, a discursive approach may provide us with a way of recognizing more complex desires and formations of ourselves. Because of this, one need not necessarily resist motherhood *per se*, in order to resist some of the particular meanings it is given in Western culture.

Hence the possibilities of a given discourse as a resource for resistance or collaboration are not fixed. This applies both between people and across time. In different contexts, discourses will operate to different ends and the conditions of particular mothers' lives might mean that discourses of a child's 'upbringing' versus a child's 'development' produce different positions. The problem with attempts to define feminist strategies of resistance around motherhood was precisely this; the meanings of a certain subject position are not identical for all women and nor can political analyses or strategies be set out for future contexts or other places. The imperative of discursive approaches to focus at the micro-level avoids such abstraction and the smoothing out of disjunctions which allow for the emergence of resistance. Similarly, theorizing the productivity of discourses in shaping as well as regulating subjectivity should allow for recognition of both the immense power of normative meanings and the possibilities for and actualities of their contestation.

Notes

1 The 'exporting' of Western ideas of 'the child' and 'their needs' to non-Western countries can be understood as displaying a remaining imperialist superiority and implicit civilizing project but, moreover, it is significant that it produces benefits for the West in terms of creating consumer needs which may then be met by the exporting country (Burman, 1994a). Campaigns around breastmilk substitutes (such as the Baby Milk Action Campaign) have shown cynical financial motives and appalling marketing strategies which exploit the fact of association with healthy (white) Western babies and how the ethnocentric universalizing of child needs can promote inappropriate or unsustainable practices.

2 *Parents* is published by EMAP Consumer Publications Ltd. Issues examined for this study were July 1992; July 1993; July 1994; June 1995.

3 *Mother and Baby* is published by EMAP Elan. Issues examined for this study were June 1993; June 1994; April 1995; June 1995.

4 This echoes the words of Dr Spock in his 'allowance' of breast-feeding in the 1957 edition of *The Commonsense Book of Childcare*; because in the end, a baby needs a 'cheerful mother more than he needs breast milk' (cf. Parmenter, 1994, p. 6).

Chapter 9

Come to the carnival: Women's humour as transgression and resistance

Brenda Goldberg

> The unruly woman is multivalent ... She can signify the radical
> Utopianism of undoing all hierarchy. She can signify pollution (dirt
> or 'matter out of place') ... As such she becomes a source of danger
> for threatening the conceptual categories which organize our
> lives ... Her ambivalence, which is the source of her oppositional
> power, is usually contained within the licence accorded to the comic
> and the carnivalesque. (Rowe, 1990, pp. 410–11)

Common women

When looking for examples of transgressive or 'unruly' women it suddenly
came to me that such women had always been there. I did not need to forage
back through history or the literature books for the 'Lady Macbeths', the
'Medusas' or the 'cackling matriarchs'; such women had been part and parcel
of a working-class culture. The women I refer to may not have constituted a
major political or revolutionary force, or even for one moment envisaged
themselves as transgressive or unruly; but they did play a significant role in the
constitution and enforcement of working-class gender norms and boundaries
while, as Davis (1965, p. 131) observes, providing a 'multivalent image',
a 'widening' of 'behavioural options' for transgressing those very same
boundaries.

Such women might be seen to have exhibited many of the features of what
will later be described as the carnivalesque. These women were the bawdy,
shrill, 'common as muck' women who lived at the margins of every working-
class community, simultaneously ostracized for their looseness but also toler-
ated as a constant source of titillating scandal. Teetering up the streets of the
1960s with their white stilettos, heavily painted faces and preposterous 'hair
dos', these were the women representing Bakhtin's (1968) 'lower bodily stratum', a lower stratum which according to the local gossips was receiving far too
much attention.

It might seem to stretch a point to credit these often fertile women with
the significance of celebratory 'becoming', decay and renewal given to the

pregnant laughing 'hags' of Bakhtin's carnival. Or even to equate such women with the pagan goddesses and the celebratory 'fecund', 'cosmic' female images promoted by some (notably French) feminist theorists. Even so, I do believe that these women deserve to be acknowledged as truly fitting for the title of 'unruly' women. That these 'types' of women have become part of British comic folklore, as immortalized within our soap operas in the shape of the 'Elsie Tanners', the 'Bet Lynchs', is evidence of their social and symbolic function, as markers of the boundaries of inclusion and exclusion, pure and unpure, fascination and disgust.

Back in the 1960s, the ribald, bawdy women of the terraced houses served to extol a dire warning to working-class girls of what would happen to them if they strayed from the path of respectable, 'classical' womanhood. You would become, like them, a 'sight', a 'spectacle' and as such deemed unfit for the company of decent women. But, on looking back, it seems as if these women's only offence was that they mocked and threatened the passive norms of femininity and the structure and stability of working-class family life. These were the women who invaded your home and took your husband. And they were allowed to inhabit the margins of working-class society precisely because they represented the repressed side of working-class womanhood, their fanta-sized bodies and lifestyle becoming the site of all that was sexual, dangerous and prohibited.

As a young working-class girl I felt an immense fascination and awe towards these cackling, 'good time', unruly women. They may have signified a 'grotesque' (Bakhtin, 1968), parodied version of the female body, but they also signified strange secret places and the promise of prohibited delights. And most enticing of all, they seemed to know how to play and have fun. And women having fun, laughing, playing, making an unashamed 'sight' and 'spec-tacle' of themselves is what this chapter is about. To try to explore and conceptualize a style of women's comedy that is neither collusive nor simply reactionary. A transgressive, dialectical comic form that simultaneously ex-poses and deconstructs the social construction of gender. A parodic form of comedy that, through its multiple imagery, problematizes and transgresses the ideological gender boundaries and binary oppositions that serve to contain and represent women within neat identity roles and stereotypical categories. My reasons for wanting to do this arise from both my position as a feminist and my interest in humour as a 'power' discourse (that has historically often been used to ridicule and suppress women) and also as a possible means of resistance.

One of the most immediate and frustrating concerns for a feminist re-searching humour is the relative lack of female humour (in the public sphere). Or, where it does exist, it is often self-derogatory and therefore defensive in character. These are issues which may seem to be reflected within feminist politics, as even to the favourable observer it might appear that feminism and feminists in the past have often seemed overly intense and lacking a sense of humour. Some of this perception no doubt arises from the political advantage to be gained from casting feminists in this dour mode, both because humourless people are regarded as aggressive and unreasonable and also as Lavery (in Banks and Swift, 1987, p. 215) states, 'Humour is a weapon and if we say that women are not funny, they can't use that weapon.' Some of our lack of confidence in using humour arises because historically women have not been positioned as the 'jokers', the initiators of humour within our Western culture and it would be naïve to suppose that we could just shrug off our public exclusion from such a powerful, masculine discourse to uncover some dormant, 'natural' form of feminine wit. This is not to imply that women have no potential for comedy, or do not express humour within the private sphere. Rather, public performances of comedy have become synonymous with high visibility, 'spectacle' and mastery and thus defined as outside the female role.

Some of our reluctance (if I may so generalize) in deploying humour no doubt also arises from the perceived trivializing effects of humour and the serious and often arduous nature of the feminist project; a sustained campaign against entrenched misogyny and oppressive practices that has left feminists with arguably little to feel they can laugh about. In a culture that has assigned women as the 'laughable' (Barreca, 1988), the butt of the joke, the very antithesis of humour, it is hard for women to transcend this public perception to know how to use humour. If women's public expression of humour is just not perceived as funny it becomes problematic how to use it in a politically persuasive, creative way.

However, as comediennes increasingly and successfully invade the public male comic domain, the time might be ripe for feminists to throw off their past seriousness and adopt a playful, irreverent attitude as an alternative form of feminist resistance. In the past, feminism's commitment to both deconstruction and identity politics has been a necessary part in the history of feminist politics. But such strategies may often have functioned in their extreme form to simply reproduce the social categorizations and the victimized status we have been trying to escape. In our enthusiastic appropriation of deconstructionist and post-structuralist perspectives (myself included), we may have become so engrossed in theorizing women's silence and exclusion from patriarchal culture and language that we have done more to publicize women's 'lack', women's status as 'object', 'Other', than either Lacan or Freud ever did. In our eagerness to fill this 'lack' and in our search for a positive feminine identity we may have often simply interpreted plurality of identity to mean the need for an endless list of alternative unified, female identities, rather than questioning the possibility of any stable, feminine identity; until, as Butler suggests, the obligatory 'embarrassed, etc.' that has become such a feature of such lists simply serves as a 'sign of exhaustion'. 'It is the *supplement*, the excess that necessarily accompanies any effort to posit identity once and for all' (Butler, 1990b, p. 143).

Thus, looking back somewhat irreverently, feminism has had its own comic moments. In our efforts to evade female stereotypes and degrading imagery we have often become stuck between divisive and irresolvable debates surrounding the political merits of essentialism versus anti-essentialism. We have been rendered paranoid and politically immobilized by the need to stress the plurality of feminine identities while not invalidating women as a politically viable group. We had to come in from the margins but not be incorporated, to achieve academic status but not be engulfed by academia, to aspire for powerful positions but not to wield power. Thus our resistance so far has often seemed defensive and still self-conscious of and controlled by patriarchal discourse. In our desire not to duplicate oppressive, patriarchal practices and to evade the degrading images that have legitimatized women's oppression, we find we have few places left to go. And as we try to reinvent or rediscover ourselves we often find that a change in boundaries or identity does not of necessity lead to social change. The ruling culture 'watches its margins' and a shift in female boundaries can merely bring about new male mutations, such as the sensitive man, leaving the power structure, and the hegemony of the new male identity, intact and unchanged.

So it would seem that it is not simply enough just to expose ideological discourse or construct new identities; we need to challenge Western concepts of identity and subjectivity themselves. This entails an analysis of how such concepts are constituted and reproduced through a patriarchal discourse, linked to a scientific/medical discourse that depends on and fetishizes difference. So it is argued that we need to devise ways not just to radically redefine the gender boundaries, but to challenge and disrupt the very nature of binary structures themselves.

Given this challenge, perhaps the only form of resistance left for feminists is to parody, laugh at, play and have fun with the very stereotypes that have ruled women's lives. In *Gender Trouble* Judith Butler (1990b) asks the question 'what possibilities of recirculation exist? What possibilities of doing gender repeat and displace through hyperbole, dissonance, internal confusion, and proliferation the very constructs by which they are mobilised?' Butler's answer to this question is the adoption of a 'disruptive' (p. 139) and 'truly troubling' parodic form. A 'parodic repetition' that 'reveals the original to be nothing other than a parody of the idea of the natural' (1990b, pp. 30–1). It is possible that such a parodic form might already exist in the form of the carnivalesque and the 'unruly' woman.

Carnival humour

The carnival and its folk humour was a prominent feature of the popular culture of the Europe of the Middle Ages. These times of feasts and spectacle were opportunities for the common people of the marketplace to suspend their normal activities and break free from the inhibitions and social restrictions imposed by the ruling classes. These local celebrations provided a temporary respite from social hierarchies and inequality, where the folk as a collective body could transgress rules of social propriety by posing the 'grotesque realism' (Bakhtin, 1968) of their over-physical, too sexual, polluted bodies; the bulging, protruding, crude and licentious body of the 'lower bodily stratum', against the 'classical' body and the pious, oppressive, rational idealism of the state. The grotesque body of the people was symbolic of a universal, earthy body, a body of ambivalent, polymorphous sexuality and dual significance, symbolizing birth and death, decay and renewal. Thus the grotesque body represented a body both real and Utopian, a body still in the state of 'becoming'; at ease with its surroundings and its own fleshy materiality. 'In the world of carnival the awareness of the people's immortality is combined with the realisation that established authority and truth are relative' (Bakhtin, 1968, p. 10).

In essence carnival became occasions where the unofficial discourse of the people met in dialogical, binary opposition with official discourse. It was, in effect, a confrontation of the body/mind, nature/culture, non-human/human oppositions. Where the classical body of the ruling classes was placed in uneasy face-to-face conflict with its own displaced and externalized 'Other', its repressed underside, its own excluded 'filth' (Bakhtin, 1968; Kristeva, 1982).

Folk humour took the form of travesty and parody, negation and inversion, whereby the pretensions of the ruling classes were degraded and ridiculed and social hierarchies ritually debunked through a series of mock 'crownings and uncrownings', 'the clown versus serious ceremonial', 'parodies versus high ideology' (Bakhtin, 1968, p. 22). The subversive power of carnival lay in its ability to deal at both the levels of fantasy and the real and in its ability to juxtapose and throw into chaos the very binary oppositions that functioned to maintain (through exclusion) ruling-class identity and power. As stated by Eagleton (1981, p. 149), carnival acted as a 'kind of fiction: a temporary retextualizing of the social formation' that functioned to expose its 'fictive foundations'.

Thus it is at the dialogical interchange, the meeting of the two discourses, the two bodies, the 'grotesque' against the 'classical', that meaning becomes displaced, flipped out of context by its contrasting image, producing what Eagleton (1989, p. 185) calls 'estrangement effects'. Here the familiar is made strange, the mundane suspect, producing a paradox of uncertainty in which accepted truths are reduced to the pompous and the comic and the imaginary stability of the body itself is returned to its fragmentary and sexual origins. As Eagleton (1981, p. 150) comments, 'The return of discourse to this sensuous root is nowhere more evident than in laughter itself, an enunciation that springs straight from the body's libidinal depths.'

It may seem a far cry from those images of the 'common' women of the terraces to the carnivalesque images of Bakhtin's theory, one which according to Stallybrass and White (1986, p. 192) has been enthusiastically appropriated by academia with often suspiciously idealistic and nostalgic results. As they observe, the celebration and appropriation of carnival by the middle classes, its fetishization and idealization of the lower orders and popular culture, has often merely served to re-endorse the splitting of high and low culture, thus strengthening, yet again, middle-class identity.

Bakhtin himself has often been accused of essentializing and idealizing carnival and the body of the people, but according to Holquist (in Bakhtin, 1968, p. xix), Bakhtin's sudden appropriation of carnival was politically motivated as a response to Stalinism. Bakhtin's celebration of the folk body and culture was posed in direct confrontation to the idealization of the working classes being peddled by the Stalinist State. In a similar hegemonic practice, our Western patriarchal culture has also sought to homogenize the category 'woman' and has perpetuated naturalized ideals of femininity as a way of legitimating women's oppression and their exclusion from the professional and cultural spheres.

When seen in this context, a reappropriation of carnival imagery does not have to mean a return to an essentialization or romanticism of the female body. On the contrary, we can use this to avoid such categorization. The essence of carnival is its emphasis on the crossing of boundaries, to avoid the binary oppositions that proliferate in official Western discourse. Transgressing boundaries does not mean to trade one identity for another; it means to confuse the boundaries so that no new easy binary oppositions can be constructed. Thus carnival imagery and humour invite a return to a body of communal action, to a reappropriation of a hedonistic, guiltless state that celebrates diversity and multiple subjectivity: to a celebration of jouissance, laughter, sexual diversity and pleasure for their own sake. Within this framework, the laughing woman, the 'unruly' woman, becomes a powerful woman, a 'prototype of woman as subject' (Rowe, 1990, p. 410).

Masquerade, carnival and the body

Masquerade

It might seem ironic that in trying to formulate a comedic form of resistance, I am advocating a return to the female body, one which in its idealized form signifies for many women the very site of their oppression. Thus the 'politic problem' becomes, as Eagleton (1989, p. 184) states, 'to know how to subvert the State's lying romantic idealism without lapsing into a version of its own lethal levelling'.

One such way might be through the concept of masquerade, as originally formulated by Joan Riviere (1929), in her paper 'Womanliness as a masquerade'. Within the masquerade, femininity becomes a parody, a performative act, in which women don the characteristics and mannerisms of femininity as a façade, a defence against an inherent masculinity and in response to the dictates and desires of a masculine culture. As such, there is no 'authentic' feminine identity. The 'mime' of femininity that women enact merely copies a copy of which there is no original (Butler, 1990b). As Heath (1986, p. 49) puts it, 'to be a woman is to dissimulate a fundamental masculinity, femininity is that dissimulation'.

Newton (1972), cited in Butler, 1990b, p. 137, uses the concept of masquerade or 'impersonation' as a means of explaining the subversive effects of drag acts as a form of 'double inversion', a clash of conflicting imagery and discourse which confuses our very senses as to any supposed relationship between body and gender: 'At its most complex, [drag] is a double inversion that says "appearance is an illusion". Drag says "my 'outside' appearance is feminine, but my essence 'inside' is masculine". At the same time it symbolizes the opposite inversion; "my appearance 'outside' is masculine but my essence 'inside' is feminine" ' (Newton, 1972, p. 103, cited in Butler, 1990b, p. 137). A performance which according to Butler (1990b, p. 137), 'fully subverts the distinction between inner and outer psychic space and effectively mocks both the expressive model of gender and the notion of a true gender identity'. For similar reasons Butler locates a parallel ambivalence in the cross-dressing practiced by some butch/femme lesbian couples, while according to Heath (1986), Hollywood and the film industry have founded an empire on the mimetic performances of such female stars as Dietrich and Garbo. 'Garbo "got into drag" whenever she took some heavy glamour part, whenever she melted in or out of a man's arms, whenever she simply let that heavenly-flexed neck . . . bear the weight of her thrown-back head . . . How resplendent seems the art of acting! It is all *impersonation*, whether the sex underneath is true or not' (Parker Tyler, quoted in Butler, 1990b, p. 128).

However, the concept of masquerade is problematic in various respects: it seems to displace womanliness only to replace it with an inherent masculinity; thus in many ways it simply rearticulates many of the themes of patriarchal and medical/psychological discourse where the masculine becomes the normal, the feminine the pathological (and the deceitful). Even if we accept that the notion of femininity, as a performative act, may have resonance for women, we are still left with the problem of what the mask – the disguise – is supposed to be disguising. So we get caught within a tautology from which even Riviere found it impossible to extricate herself.

Moreover, it is difficult to appreciate the transgressive potential of such parodic forms when they are still shackled to, and reproductive of, the gender categories promoted and valued by Western culture. By simply parodying fetishized forms of femininity they run the risk of becoming fetishized objects, fantasy vehicles themselves; a fate which befell Dietrich and Garbo, whose subversive attempts were no doubt missed by most movie audiences.

So concepts such as 'femininity as masquerade' (as in their original and essentialistic formulation) tend to be unhelpful to women, showing themselves as still harnessed to the either/or dualisms about gender that operate in our culture, one which still relates authenticity and thus value to some biological or 'natural' state. To articulate the construction of subjectivity and gender through cultural and discursive practices does not invalidate authenticity or lived experience. It merely questions the unproblematic adoption of any unified, stable subject and gender identity. Within such a framework we are constituted through a multitude of contradictory discourses, subject and gender positionings, any of which might become articulated or repressed depending on the social context, the demands and the taboos, operating within a culture at any given time. Problems of oppression occur when society seeks to deny our diversity of being through the imposition of rigid homogenous social categories. In other words, when it insists we don the masquerade and limit our repertoire to a particular rendition of self.

Carnival

It is possible that the concept of masquerade, as a performative act, becomes useful if incorporated within a carnivalesque framework. Through its kaleidoscope of conflicting imagery, carnival parodies the homogenizing tendencies of official discourse; and through exaggeration, hyperbole and inversion exposes its reductionist, repressive and ideological foundations. Here, too, it has been argued that most parody is ultimately conformist, as even by parodic repetition it merely rearticulates and reproduces the object it supposes to mock. Within these terms carnival itself has been described as a form of 'licensed . . . blow off', by which the authorities have allowed public demonstrations as a means of controlling public unrest and anger (Eagleton, 1981, p. 148). Ultimately, debates about the inherent subversiveness of carnival prove redundant. As Stallybrass and White (1986, p. 14) state, what is important is how 'Given the presence of sharpened political antagonism, it [carnival] may often act as catalyst and site of actual and symbolic struggle.'

Therefore whether carnival is transgressive or not will depend on a combination of factors: the political group (both Stallybrass and White, 1986, and Eagleton, 1989, acknowledge that only oppressed groups can use carnival transformatively), the political context and political readiness. Since women undoubtedly qualify as a marginalized group this suggests carnival may be a possible political strategy.

But one of the most convincing arguments for the adoption of carnival or carnival humour is that it is feared. Throughout history – indeed, in Bakhtin's Stalinist Russia – authorities alarmed by such spectacles of collective action have either sought to repress it or incorporate it under the banner of officially organized pageantry (Bakhtin, 1968). That women have historically been excluded as initiators of humour and defined as having no sense of humour is also evidence of humour as a feared and powerful discourse. As stated by Gagnier (in Barreca, 1988, p. 137) 'men fear women's humour for much the same reason that they fear women's sexual freedom – because they encourage women's aggression and promiscuity and thus disrupt the social order . . . therefore men desire to control women's humour just as they desire to control women's sexuality.'

Brenda Goldberg

The body

One of the reasons why the body (and thus the female body) has gained such obsessive importance as a site of conflict is because of its status as an original signifier: the earliest site of classification and division. The semiology of the body as an ideologically discursive form has become descriptive and prescriptive of both Western social structure and Western concepts of subjectivity and identity. The symbolism inscribed upon the classical body, perhaps exemplified in Rodin's sculpture *The Thinker*, become elements associated with 'high' culture and a notion of the subject as masculine, rational, closed and monumentally centred; against an expelled and degraded (and by association female) 'grotesque' body symbolizing through its open orifices, its secretions, its 'expelled filth' (Kristeva, 1982), mortality, impurity, uncontrollable sexuality and ambivalence of 'being'.

So at the conscious level the carnivalesque body has been degraded and subordinated to symbolic, official language and its subject forms. But as a repressed discourse located within and through the body, it continues to structure all local and global relations (Stallybrass and White, 1986). To accept the body and its inscriptions as the site of the conflict is not to invest the body or woman as one of its main sites of representation with any essential status or signification. It is merely to contest an official structure that maintains its identity and its claim to power through an externalization and psychic distancing of the body and its feared associations on to other sites and groups. Here the carnival and the 'grotesque' body as a locus of disgust and desire did not disappear with the decline of carnival activity in public life. It merely changed its site: moved from the public and external sphere to the private, repressed domain. The activity and manifestations of that repressed discourse and its negative associations of filth and pollution continue to structure and express themselves through all aspects of cultural life.

A horror story

Barbara Creed (1987) explores how Western culture attempts to articulate and resolve its terror of the carnivalized, maternal body through the medium of the horror story. A 'grotesque', 'monstrous', castrating maternal body which is perceived to always threaten to transgress its own boundaries; to re-engulf its victims back into a psychotic, undifferentiated state. According to Creed, it is through its symbolic imagery that the horror story expresses these fears of 're-incorporation', 'fusion' and 'dissolution' (pp. 61–3). Within horror stories, ambivalent feelings of fear and desire are ritually exorcized through the storyline, when the maternal body represented in such forms, as the 'toothed vagina' (the fanged monster in *Alien* and *Aliens*), or the claustrophobic, 'pulsating' womb cave (*Aliens*, *Dracula*) (Creed, 1987, p. 63), is vanquished and expelled along with the themes of blood, excrement and psychotic death ('*Night of the Living Dead*', *Zombies*).

That these forms of exorcism, or 'cleansing rituals', are not just confined to the genre of the horror movie, but are re-enacted within everyday life is apparent in 'dramas' such as Greenham Common. Here, the response to the demonstrating women assumed a significance that was out of all proportion to the threat the women posed. Even the military establishment (the male, classical, military body) seemed to view the women as almost as dangerous as the armaments themselves. Defined as a monstrous, female invading force, the women were seen to threaten territorial, gender and power boundaries, thereby evoking 'scapegoating carnivalesque ritual', such as the smearing of blood and excrement on their tents, 'a rowdy form of crowd behaviour often used against "unruly" women' as 'an overt reminder of patriarchal dominance' (Stallybrass and White, 1986, p. 24). Within this instance we see many of the same images and themes identified by Creed in her analysis of the horror film; the same attempts to safeguard a male, rational subject from the encroachment of a castrating, maternal body.

Another horror story

We can make analogies between scientific discourse and the horror story not only in a metaphorical but a literal sense. The history of rationality is strewn with its own tales of horror in the treatment of those it has designated as 'Other', 'monstrous', and pathological in their difference (also see Chapters 5 and 6 in this volume). As Stallybrass and White (1986, pp. 22–3) comment: 'Foucault's concentration upon the contained outsiders-who-make-the-insiders-insiders (the mad, the criminal, the sick, the unruly, the sexually transgressive) reveals just how far these outsiders are constructed by the dominant culture in terms of the grotesque body.'

Past medical and psychological abuse of the transgressive, 'unruly' woman, through such medical procedures as clitoredectomy and hysterectomy (Ussher, 1991) have all been legitimatized within the framework of a rational, male discourse that sought to locate and expel through the 'alien' body of the grotesque feminine its own fears which it had inscribed on to those bodies. These mutilating practices were a direct attempt to control women's latent threat, their uncontrollable sexuality through a control of their bodily functions and wastes (their blood and filth); through ritualized medical expellation (surgical removal) and menstruation taboos. Such 'cleansing' efforts sought to rehabilitate the 'unruly' women, the sexually promiscuous, the disobedient wife and the hysteric back within the safe confines of the sexually passive, the domestic and the pure. But, as Creed points out, the negative images and associations of the 'grotesque' body and the 'monstrous feminine' are those that a male culture has retroactively conferred on the maternal space and the pre-Oedipal mother. Its negative significance or threat is the response of a patriarchal culture that prizes order and rationality above all else and perceives in the feminine a threat to that order.

Brenda Goldberg

So the problem becomes how to conceptualize a form of resistance to an institutionalized patriarchy which has a positive investment in maintaining and fetishizing difference. This is because it needs that very difference, that 'Other', that repository of all it rejects (and secretly covets) to maintain its own identity and position of power. How do we, as the group 'woman', reason with a rational, ideological discourse whose very motivations are based on fear and unreason themselves?

Humour and the unruly woman

The appropriation of carnival humour as a transgressive form of women's rebellion and as a strategy for feminist politics is not a new idea. According to Rowe (1990, p. 410) the transgressive female has had a long, if marginalized, career; has taunted and been 'making a spectacle' of herself throughout history, breaking social and gender boundaries, signifying 'sexual inversion', 'multivariance' and 'pollution'.

Using the comedy show *Roseanne*, and the 'character' and person of 'Roseanne' as an example, Rowe demonstrates the power of the unruly woman to 'demystify', or put into question feminine stereotypes. Rowe contends that the 'person' and 'character' of 'Roseanne' both fascinates and repels. This ambivalence has been reflected in both the popularity of the show and the malice of the press who have often homed in on the supposed decadence of Roseanne's character, body and lifestyle. Rowe argues that the show is subversive for various reasons. First because it problematizes the relationship between fiction and reality, as 'Roseanne' embodies all three elements of author, 'character' and actual person. This also means that by female standards she has considerable control as to how she is represented within the show in terms of subjectivity and desire. Rowe suggests that the most subversive attributes of the 'unruly' woman, as epitomized by 'Roseanne', are ambivalence and excess. So in a world where women are often relegated to a marginal, small, silent and powerless position, the unruly woman is just too much of everything; she's 'too fat, too mouthy, too old, too dirty . . . too sexual' (Rowe, 1990, p. 410). She takes up too much space, laughs too loudly, 'picks her nose' and 'farts' and flaunts her sensuality in a manner expressing both relish and unselfconscious delight. Her ambiguity and our ambivalent envy (as well as disgust) stems from her capacity to adopt conflicting subject positions, to freely move across and inhabit the borders of what is permissible and prohibited, so throwing into disarray accepted gender norms, challenging their 'naturalness' and inevitability.

As Rowe states, 'Roseanne's' subversive power emanates through her body. It is the bawdy, parodic, mocking laughing body of carnival, an uninhibited body which denies male fantasy and desire and 'moons' at patriarchal dictates of what women should be. 'Her body epitomizes the grotesque body of Bakhtin, the body which exaggerates its processes, its bulges and

162

orifices, rather than concealing them as the monumental, static "classical" or "bourgeois" body does' (Rowe, 1990, p. 413).

Hysterically funny women

One of the most obvious instances of carnivalesque action is that of the British Women's Suffrage Movement. Although there is much literature relating Bakhtin's carnival to feminist politics, there are surprisingly few connections to the suffragettes. This may be because the suffrage movement was primarily a middle-class venture. However, as a working-class woman myself, I think this view tends to dismiss the extra determination required of the working-class women who did manage to get involved. And at the level of patriarchy, all women could in their various roles be conceived as suffering the exploitation and status of the proletariat. So despite this class conflict and without romanticizing the issue, this surely still has to be one of the most significant episodes of female, collective political action in which many of the elements of carnival and carnival humour are to be seen.

Although the suffrage campaign was ostensibly a political movement about women getting the vote, the terms of the debate again centred around the possession and control of the female body. In an era increasingly influenced by Darwinian theory and thus typology (character type linked to body type), as Tickner (1987, p. 151) observes 'the Victorian and Edwardian public expected to see the virtues and vices of femininity written on the body'. Given the (then as now) perceived importance of the external female form as an indicator of internal virtue, the campaign became, as Tickner states, one primarily of 'agitation by symbol' (p. 16), in which title to authorship and control of the female image became of importance to both suffragettes and anti-suffragettes alike. It was a campaign often seemingly directed and waged at the level of the repressed, with the suffragettes cast within the imagery and the imagination as an invading, monstrous 'polluting' agent, 'an influx of something dangerously, hysterically feminine' (Tickner, 1987, pp. 154–5).

Thus the campaign became a sexualized one, where humour and parody played a significant part in the propaganda promoted by both suffrage and anti-suffrage supporters. A war of classical versus grotesque imagery, with anti-suffrage cartoonists invariably exploiting public fears by portraying suffragettes in terms of the pathological, the ugly and the masculine, the lesbian and the uncaring mother. The punishment for transgression became focused again on the female body in terms of penal incarceration and force-feeding. The suffragettes were seen not only to be transgressing gender boundaries but all other binary oppositions as well. Demands for justice and equality in terms of the right to vote became translated as threats to the very fabric of Edwardian and Victorian society. As Tickner (1987, p. 170) comments, 'Woman, or rather "womanliness" was the linchpin in bourgeois ideology and a structuring category in the principal discourses of civil society (medicine, law, politics, education, the family). If woman was out of place everything was out of place.'

Given the level of antagonism against them, the suffragettes and their artists used any feminine imagery or discourse that would further their political cause. Their choice was pragmatic rather than Utopian, they 'cut their cloth according to the context in which they found themselves' (Tickner, 1987, p. 151). A plurality of images were plucked out of time and context and reproduced on placards and posters to produce a pastiche of images with little regard for historical accuracy. Because the women recognized there was no natural female identity or essence to draw on, they could only use to their best strategic advantage the intertextuality of discourses on femininity available to them at the time. The campaign therefore set out not to construct some new homogenous identity for women but to deconstruct an old one, to expose the fallacy and the fantasy of an idealized Victorian protected womanhood against the harsh reality of an exploited and unprotected female underclass. So the purpose of the campaign became 'to demythologise the dominant ideology of Edwardian femininity, to fill out its absences and exploit its contradictions', a campaign that 'used all the rhetorical devices at [its] disposal (analogy, parody, hyperbole, reversal) to impugn the motives and puncture the arguments of [its] opponents' (Tickner, 1987, p. 152).

As an example of such parody we have below what might be described in carnival terms as a dialogue between official (Figure 9.1, anti-suffrage poster) and non-official discourse (Figure 9.2, the suffrage response). Both posters can be seen to be using contrasting grotesque and classical imagery. In Figure 9.1 we see the classical, idealized version of Victorian and Edwardian womanhood foregrounded against what Tickner (1987, p. 192) terms the 'shrieking sister', the hysterical, monstrous figure of the hammer-wielding suffragette. The message is clear: 'real', desirable, feminine women do not need or desire the vote. There is also the covert threat that the vote will somehow transform ordinary women into the grotesque image. In the parodic reply produced by the suffragettes (Figure 9.2) we again see the classical female body but this time it is less sexualized, more warrior-like. And this time the female figure (a suffragette) may be seen to be protecting the 'grotesque' body of women walking abjectedly behind her.

In the true spirit of carnival humour the subversive effects of the parody only occur at the meeting point of the two discourses, at the dialogical interchange. It is at this point that contradictions between the two discourses become explicit. We have the diverse, 'realistically' portrayed, images of women (Figure 9.2) juxtaposed against the stereotypical, idealized, singular image of womanhood (Figure 9.1). The parody is effective because it contrasts two discourses: an ideological discourse that posits an idealized image of womanhood as a pivotal support for a fictitious, chivalrous, protective Victorian male identity and culture against a repressed discourse that stresses the neglect, 'expellation' and abuse of working-class women. The (explicit) political context in both posters is provided by the Houses of Parliament in the background.

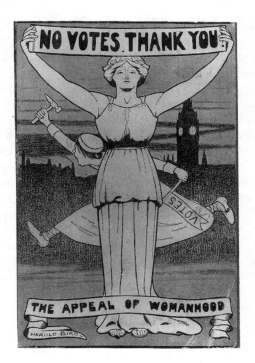

Figure 9.1 *'No Votes Thank You': designed by Harold Bird, 1912.*

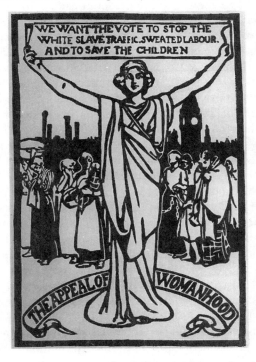

Figure 9.2 *'The Appeal of Womanhood': designed by Louise Jacobs, 1912.*

165

Elements of Bakhtin's carnival permeate all levels of the suffragette campaign. There is the collective body of 'unruly' women making a deliberate and highly visible 'sight' and 'spectacle' of themselves both through their own carnivalized activities of chaining themselves to railings and glass-breaking and within the vibrant, colourful, carnival atmosphere of the pageants and parades: 'the amazing spectacle of two miles of women – women of every class, of every profession and calling' (Lawrence, 1910, cited in Tickner, 1987, p. 55). A heterogeneous body of women from all strata of society pitted against and carnivalized by a patriarchal culture and an ideology of femininity that functioned to constrain women within a homogenous ideal of femininity that masked an underside of suppressed and exploited womanhood. An official, rational discourse that supported its arguments by 'scientific' evidence which linked differences in physiology to pathology, where 'anatomy' became 'destiny'. A discourse which (as cited by Louisa Jopling advocating the use of satire as a political tactic) decrees 'that women having no sense of humour, cannot register votes' (in Tickner, 1987, p. 34).

Monstrously funny women

It is hard to imagine such well-orchestrated instances of women's carnival collective action happening in the more politically cynical, fragmented and apathetic social climate of the 1990s, where such phrases as 'post-feminism' abound and radical forms of political action might be viewed as embarrassingly *passé* and extreme in an era where individual legal action has apparently – on paper at least – taken away the need for elaborate shows of social action. So at a time when the threat of unemployment cuts across all sectors of society and where such phrases as 'Britain as a slave economy' have become unshocking, other social and political causes might seem trivial and self-indulgent in comparison.

In a society depressed under the weight of national problems, where escapism might seem more desirable to most people than political confrontation, how might feminists engage public interest? One answer might seem to be by exploiting this need for pleasure through an escalation of female comedy through those vehicles where most people escape: the television set and the media. So shackling oneself to railings might have been effective in the 1920s, protest marches, 'love ins', going bra-less appropriate feminist action during the Utopian atmosphere of the 1960s and 1970s, an emphasis on female writing, informed debate, padded shoulders and 'superwoman', a strategy for the 1980s. On this basis it seems that persuasion through pleasure might be a suitable feminist strategy for a media-driven, pleasure-orientated, increasingly postmodern culture.

With this in mind, I should like to analyse features of one contemporary comedy TV show *Absolutely Fabulous*, which shows many of the subversive elements of the carnivalesque, taking into account that it inevitably suffers from being confined within the restrictions imposed by the popular media. Within *Absolutely Fabulous* we find many of the features of the carnivalesque and the 'unruly' woman identified by Rowe (1990) in her analysis of *Roseanne*. We have the excessive, loud, strutting, bawdy, too-sexual women represented through the bodies of the two main characters of the show, Patsy and Eddy. However, unlike the character of 'Roseanne' the subversive comic effects are not produced through any 'natural' qualities that might be attributed to the actresses' own bodies but through the obvious artifices and constructions of femininity that are inscribed on the surfaces of the female characters. Thus the overall effect becomes one of 'masquerade', or one of women 'passing' as women (see Chapter 10 in this volume), resulting in a parody of the trappings and adornments of femininity which is comic when juxtaposed against the unfeminine counter discourses also articulated through the main characters: their aggression and cruelty, their brash obscenity, their licentious lifestyles and leering faces – a parody made even more disconcerting through occasional glimpses of vulnerability, wisdom and compassion.

The 'grotesque realism' of Eddy and Patsy is made even more explicit through comparisons with the foils of 'classical' womanhood, provided by Eddy's daughter (Saffron) and Eddy's mother (Mother), both of whom are cast within more traditional, subdued feminine roles and clothes. But even these seemingly less 'monstrous', more 'normal' feminine characters are saved from cloying conventionality and uniformity as they at various times reveal their possessive jealousy and latent sexuality (Saffron) and biting, gleeful sarcasm and malice (Mother). As the show develops it becomes problematic as to which versions of femininity should be read as masquerade: the overblown, hyperbole of Eddy and Patsy, the pious sanctimony of Saffron or the prosy motherliness of Mother. It is the transparent constructions and inscriptions of femininity, belied by the underlying tensions, conflicting discourses, shifting identities of the main characters that make the show potentially subversive. This gives the characters a curious credibility, unpredictability and variability that approximates more to the complex, multiple and diverse ways that women experience other women.

Absolutely Fabulous is above all a story about female relationships; the conflicting, irrational, emotional and sexual ways in which a family of women relate to each other. Carnival posits a state of polymorphous sexuality, where the drives of the body, unhampered by sexual taboos, are free to discharge themselves through a multiplicity of objects. In *Absolutely Fabulous* the relationships between the women play around the incestuous; the desire for the mother. Roles are swopped, relationships inverted. The daughter, Saffron, takes over the maternal function but at the same time competes with Patsy, Eddy's best friend, in sibling rivalry for the recognition and possession of Eddy, the monstrous child-mother. A monstrous mother, complete with Medusa snake-like curls, manages to evade the suffocating stereotype by her inverted, hippy-style, lax model of parental care.

While mothers figure prominently within the script, male characters are noticeably absent, or where they do appear they are relegated to the margins as insignificant and transitory beings, casual encounters and couplings to be exploited and enjoyed, with little or no lasting relevance to either the script or the family of women. Thus essentially all the female characters are rendered fatherless, a trick of the 'unruly' woman, according to Stevenson (in Broe, 1987, p. 88), who by this unfathering manages to disrupt a paternal capitalist structure: 'the transgressive female introduces uncertainty into an economic system', 'promoting the biological uncertainty of paternity which vexes a patriarchal system'.

Like *Roseanne* the show also problematizes 'reality' through its adoption of carnival time. A carnival time reminiscent of the suffrage artists, with no respect for historical exactitude, importing images from other time and spatial zones through the use of flashbacks and dream sequences, taking the 'hippy' clothes, values and lifestyle of the 1960s and 1970s, as displayed on the baby-boomer bodies of Eddy and Patsy, to produce a pastiche of discordant images and discourses here in the present.

In the show the overwhelming impression becomes one of colour and vitality. Vibrant, gaudy, festive, carnival colour is reflected both in the flamboyant clothes and colourful speech of the characters, as well as in their highly emotional, dramatic posturings. It is a performance that pantomimes the stereotype of the hysteric to its limit, so managing to transcend the pathos and the victimized status of the Victorian medical model, to bypass feminist theorizings of hysteria as protest or revolt, to emerge as sheer parody and fun. The flamboyant behaviour is in line with the general flamboyant atmosphere. In the show women humourists control their own definitions of subjectivity, sensuality and visibility and write and act their own comedy, using the whole gamut of female stereotypes, both negative and positive, without any concern to portray women in a politically expedient light, a tactic that seems curiously liberating and empowering. It is women seemingly not caring any more, 'mooning' at patriarchal constructs, sending up degrading images and stereotypes, appropriating and reformulating them in their own creative, unselfconscious and irreverent way.

Absolutely Fabulous allows for no resolutions, whether feminist or otherwise. Identities and relationships shift and change so often that there is no easy way to separate or compartmentalize the characters into fixed, stable personalities or roles. There are no heroines of the piece. All the characters, both the monstrous and classical, are at various times both likeable and dislikeable in their vulnerabilities and petty foibles. As such, the show alternately entertains and frustrates, provokes and offends our sense of what femininity is or should be. We look for the expected redemption of the characters, for Eddy to become a good mother, for Patsy to settle down, but they don't respond. We look for their better side but there often just isn't one. We look for the happy endings but don't get them. We look for the caring, nurturing, passive female, but she is just not there.

Following the carnival

The new historian, the genealogist, will know what to make of this masquerade. [She] will not be too serious to enjoy it; on the contrary [she] will push the masquerade to its limits and prepare the great carnival of time where masks are constantly reappearing. Genealogy is history in the form of a concerted carnival. (Foucault, 1977b, pp. 160–1)

The history of the women's movement is full of real transgressive women who have committed social heresy, dared to cross gender and other boundaries in order to pursue personal and collective visions of a better and more equal future for women. When such women have stepped out of line, carnivalesque imagery, such as the image of the aggressive, ball-breaking feminist and 'cleansing rituals' have been brought into force in an attempt to dispel the danger: the danger of a woman 'out of place', who if left unchecked will put everything else 'out of place'. That such women, past and present, have provoked such extreme and hostile reactions is itself a sign of their transformative potential. What incites fear and ridicule is often truly dangerous in terms of its threat to existing power and social structures.

However, by my celebration of carnival and 'unruly' women I am not suggesting that we, to follow 'Roseanne's' example, should take to picking our noses and farting in public places as signs of our subversive power and 'subject' status (although why not?). More that we should adopt the spirit of carnival and carnival humour. There is no more dangerous and powerful image than that of a woman who laughs, mocks and travesties the bonds that are designed to bind her. Who no longer feels that she has to avoid negative, female images, but dons those negative images with derision and relish, knowing that she is transgressing boundaries, offending patriarchal sensitivities, undermining masculine identities and revelling in the fact.

When we as women stop looking over our shoulders in order to parry the next patriarchal attack, when we cease as de Lauretis (1989) suggests to cast ourselves in this victim's role and no longer care whether we incite masculine approval or disapproval, is when we might say we have become 'subjects'. So we need to conceptualize power not so much about how we as women are represented, but in terms of having the power and the social confidence to create and impose our own definitions of subjectivity and sexuality. As Bourdieu (in Rowe, 1990, p. 414) states, to adopt 'a sort of indifference to the objectifying gaze of others which neutralizes its power ... appropriates its appropriation'. Within this framework, making a 'spectacle' of yourself can be powerful if you chose to do it when you are the 'subject' and creator of your own representation and visibility.

Chapter 10

The rhetorics of gender identity clinics: Transsexuals and other boundary objects

Ángel Juan Gordo López

This final chapter analyses the rhetorics of gender identity clinics in the light of a discursive interpretation of the notion of 'boundary objects'. We suggest this notion can contribute to other relational understandings of the nets of psychology, including complex relationships between (sexual) bodies and technologies of gender. We borrow some conceptual developments from ethnographic studies and the sociology of scientific knowledge to textualize *technologies of gender* in the frame of discursive-analytical work. In the first part we examine regulatory practices within gender identity clinics: that is, clinics attended by people who wish to change sex. We discuss how different groups of practitioners are coordinated through constituting their 'clients' as *boundary objects* and how these objects, informed by wider social discourses, are regulated and constructed through stereotyped and binary sexual and gender divisions. By this process and ostensibly to facilitate transsexuals' social adjustment, we show how ambiguities and doubts about gender and sexuality, multiple gender positions, biographies and desires are silenced. In the second half we outline a more progressive analysis of boundary objects in relation to the possibilities and tensions existing within the project of sex/gender change as performed within gender identity clinics. In this our narrative moves on to illustrate the mutual and reciprocal relationships between the dynamics of resistance and regulation. The chapter ends by commenting on other instances of sexually ambiguous positions (e.g. 'Boys from Brazil') and advertisements of sex transformation shops in the UK. These highlight questions of agency, class and new forms of gender and subjectivities possible within the late capitalist market, of which gender identity clinics are simply one site of regulation and/or resistance.

Etymological and technological concerns

The term 'transsexualism' would not be available in our linguistic repertoire and medical dictionaries without the surgical techniques originally applied to repair nature's sexual 'mistakes' (such as hermaphrodites – people exhibiting both male and female genitalia) at the John Hopkins Hospital in the USA in the second half of this century. Surgical techniques and technologies developed in the context of medical practices made it possible for us to use this word to refer to those people, who not long ago were diagnosed as having sexual and mental disturbances. Technologies and the social conditions which reshape their (discursive) design and development allowed sex-changes which in turn work to harmonize relationships between gender identities, bodies and medical discourses.

These conceptual and material issues take practical form with the question: Why do people who want to change sex have to pass through intensive counselling if they do not really suffer, as medical-psychological research in the field indicates, any more psychological deviance than the rest of the population? Another etymological consideration may help to elucidate this question. As Shapiro (1991) notes, it is significant that practitioners involved in sex-change programmes in gender identity clinics refer to these practices as 'sex change reassignment' rather than 'gender reassignment'. According to medical-psychological assumptions, these people are supposed to already have a gender identity formed in the course of past experience, but one which is discordant with their bodies (or gender *dysphoria*).

In this chapter we pose the following questions: Is not really gender identity constructed within these gender identity clinics (hereafter GICs) by means of day-to-day regulations and acts, rather than being stable after some (early developmental) stages delimited by such notions as a 'trial period'? Do GICs, their rhetorics, technologies and expert knowledges play the role of 'gender inspectors' or institutionalized second Oedipal figures? (Gordo-López, 1994).

These sorts of questions within the context of this book and in particular this final section cannot be answered without considering, first, how the *technologies of gender* prolong stereotyped views of gender identity in these clinical settings which are informed by dominant sexual policies; and, second, without adopting a discursive approach sensitive to the functioning of GICs and their coordination of different actors participating in them (including their technologies). This chapter starts by introducing the notion of boundary object to examine the way these different actors and bodies of knowledge (discourses) and technologies (discursive hardware) become coordinated. This conceptual device of the boundary object helps to highlight both regulatory sexual policies and strategies of resistance that are performed within GICs. It is in the border zones between the symbolic/material, relation/commodity and global/local dualisms where the different regulatory and empowering interpretations of boundary objects will be located. This is because, as has been exemplified throughout this book, there is no regulation without resistance, or empowerment without constraints (Foucault, 1980a, 1992; de Lauretis, 1989).

Reframing the notion of boundary objects in a discursive approach

A main feature of the discourse analytic approach adopted here is the study of practices in their context of occurrence. We develop a perspective that emphasizes the multiple possibilities both suppressed and mobilized by the performance of these practices. Examining their performative dimension allows us to highlight the way these practices prolong and/or subvert the textualities which enable their occurrence and, in doing so, dis/locate institutional boundaries while exploring their variability and functional effects (Burman and Parker, 1993).

Institutions and the discourses that regulate their practices allow different positions for people within them. Some post-structuralist feminist research, which also informs the discursive approach applied here and in different ways in some of the previous chapters (Chapters 6, 8 and 9), maintains that multiple and dispersed experiences cannot always be gathered together under common identities and predefined political agendas (de Lauretis, 1989; Butler, 1990b, 1992; Haraway, 1991; Bondi, 1993; Burman, 1994b). However, as we argue earlier (Chapters 8 and 9), social dynamics are performed, prolonged and renewed in local settings in a systematic rather than random way in relation to specific discourses and practices.

The notion of boundary object applied here draws on the studies by Star and Griesemer (1989) and in particular their study of the history of a natural history science museum. These authors put forward the concept of boundary object to analyse the ways institutions handle and restrict variety. In their study of the history of a natural history science museum, Star and Griesemer (1989) elucidate the way participants from different social worlds, including professional scientists, amateur naturalists, patrons, administrators and scientific findings become coordinated, despite their disparate characters. Their ideas can be summarized in the form of three proposals. First, boundary objects can be both material (for example a database, protocols for gathering and analysing different data, or in the context of this chapter, surgical advances) or conceptual (for example gender stereotypes). As the authors indicate: 'Boundary Objects . . . are both plastic enough to adapt to local needs and the constraints of the several parties employing them, yet robust enough to maintain a common identity accross sites . . . The creation and management of boundary objects is a key process in developing and maintaining coherence across intersecting social worlds' (Star and Griesemer, 1989, p. 393).

Second, boundary objects coordinate people, knowledge and technologies over time and space. They are helpful in analysing the ways interdisciplinary teams, knowledges and procedures function together in institutional settings (such as GICs). For example, in the context of our analysis, we can apply this notion to the experimental condition to which subjects are exposed while answering a gender identity questionnaire. This scientific procedure serves to create new associations between the expert, the psychometric procedure, the attribution of gender personality attributes, individuals' actions and manageable and predictable portrayals of the self by means of available categories. Third, boundary objects are also valuable devices for analysing the way institutions handle and restrict variety (e.g. definitions of transsexualism and/or gender) (based on Star and Griesemer, 1989).

Recently, Yoneyama and Markussen (1993), in the context of ethno-graphic studies in work settings, view timetables as boundary objects. Time-tables are utilized as meeting points for different kinds of understandings of an organizational setting (Robinson, 1993). Another example of boundary objects proposed by Robinson (1993), in the context of computer supported cooperative work (CSCW), is the construction of a set of documents in a hospital. Robinson discusses the construction of a database for the coordination of hospital information and activities. The database supports and coordinates many users (receptionist, nurses, surgeons, administrators, book-keepers) enabling interchanges (patient information, medicines and symp-toms, diagnoses, patient flow) from different perspectives and from different locations and times (Robinson, 1993).

The concept of boundary object developed in this chapter explores the ways in which various actors (including sexual stereotypes, gender positions, scientific disciplines, legal regulations and texts extracted from the mass me-dia) are coordinated. The notion of 'actor' here draws on actor network theory (ANT) – mainly associated with the work by Latour (1986) and Callon (1991) – and spans both human and non-human agencies. In contrast to terms such as 'personality', 'identity', 'self-concept' or 'social representations', actor network theorists speak about agencies. These are continuously defined and redefined by associations of (human and non-human) actors. Thus ANT con-ceives of society and agency as the result of heterogeneous and unpredictable interactions between actors (Michael, 1994). In the course of these interac-tions actors negotiate their relationships, their 'identities' and definitions of reality (including definitions of gender). This understanding entails that social agencies and individuals' agencies within these are mutually constructed and permanently exposed to transformations. These transformations may or may not survive relationships and knowledge depending on the status of associa-tions between the different actors at different times. This framework will contribute here to a performative and discursive analysis of the rhetorics of GICs (Gordo López, 1995a).

Before moving on to discussing the sexual discourses and their articula-tion in GICs by means of boundary objects, an example will show how these mediators 'have different meanings in different social worlds, but their struc-ture is common enough to more than one world to make them recognizable' (Star and Griesemer, 1989, p. 393).

As Stone (1991, p. 291) indicates, Benjamin's (1966) book was the 're-searchers' standard reference and the source to assess the adequacy of trans-sexual 'candidates' behavioural profiles. Benjamin's (1966) book can be considered a concrete boundary object in so far as it coordinated many prac-tices and discourses across sites. It was used by different actors with disparate effects. For instance, it was also accessible to the transsexual community who therefore came to know how to perform in order to pass the test. Therefore the book was a concrete boundary object. It coordinated different actors. Among these, as will be more fully explained below, we can mention human actors including doctors, psychologists, counsellors, surgeons and people who feel unhappy with their biological sex, and other non-human actors such as technical advances in surgery, medical discourses and medical sources on transsexualism, research fundings and mass media opinion.

Sexual discourses, gender technologies and boundary objects

In his attempt to unravel the economy of bodies and pleasures, Foucault (1985) documents the case of the French hermaphrodite, Herculine Barbin. In the eighteenth century Herculine was assigned the sex of 'female' at birth. Later, in her twenties, she was allowed to shift to the category 'male'. Foucault (1979a) illustrates the way that biomedical and legal discourses of that century, as well as now, were not open to negotiating the possibility of having both sexes in a single body. Moreover, Foucault (1985) develops this analysis suggesting that currently sexuality is represented as a well-formed identity rather than shaped by actions and contexts, including legal discourses. As Varela indicates, these discourses maintain 'polymorphous and organized power technologies in which doctors, psychiatrists and psychologists play a part ... Their interventions and knowledges allow ... the convergence of disciplinary power and biopower in which sex becomes a political target of maximum priority' (Varela, 1994, p. 15: my translation). Thus sexuality became the decisive arena for the production of unitary identities in order to account for manageable representations of the (sexual) *self* (Butler, 1990b; Varela, 1994).

We argue that similar discourses regarding sexual reassignment are currently perpetuated by GICs. We suggest that the functioning of GICs can be identified by analysing their coordination by means of relational devices such as boundary objects. Before this we need to introduce some aspects of the history of transsexualism.

Some notes on the biomedical history of transsexualism

The history of transsexualism has its orgins in the USA in the second half of this century at Johns Hopkins Hospital where surgical techniques were applied to hermaphrodites. Transsexualism was for a long time portrayed as a sexual disturbance by biomedical and psychological research (Money, 1955; Stoller, 1968, 1975; Green, 1987). The common belief expressed in the media, medical and popular practices, as reflected by the most successful and common argument held by those applicants who could afford the sex-change, was that there was an inherent contradiction between their 'bodies' and their 'minds'. However, sex-change operations in the 1970s became less popular in the USA after some research affirmed that post-operational transsexuals were not happier citizens (Vincent, 1993, p. 6). So the goal of these practices, defined as improving psychological wellbeing, was not fulfilled.

By means of incorporating psychological theories of gender development and early socialization, this biomedical tradition presented itself as having a liberal approach toward sexuality. However, stereotyped and androcentric values underlie Hopkins' tradition. It is significant that this trend of research includes examinations of whether or not wearing the opposite sex's clothes increases sexual arousal. This is taken as an important factor for the selection of candidates for sex-change operations. As Garber (1992) notes, Stoller (1968) and associated workers maintain descriptions which reflect male doctors' ideas of what it is to be a woman. The following is a transcript retrospectively constructed by Richard Green ('RG') of a clinical interview between himself, a doctor and psychologist, and his client, 'Todd', in the process of deciding about sex reassignment:

RG: When you think about dressing as a woman, is that a sexual turn-on for you? Does that give you an erection?

Todd: No. And I don't need to dress like a woman to feel like a woman . . .

RG: But you'd feel more comfortable if you were dressed as one?

Todd: I wouldn't always go around dressed like one, like all made up or anything. It's just that I'd feel free that I could if I wanted. I'd probably still wear jeans because I like jeans. And I'd probably even keep my hair short, too. I don't like long hair. I'd keep my nails long.

RG: So, what part is important for such a drastic change? (Taken from Green, 1987, p. 125)

Doctor Green takes for granted the fetishistic aspect of clothing and identifies it with the wish to *become* a woman (rather than attraction *to* her). Paradoxically, the erection, signifying male sexual arousal, is taken as an indication of Todd's wish to become a woman: that is, to have the body of, and experience the desire of, a woman. Todd's persistent denial of fulfilling stereotyped views of a 'real woman' during his/her sex change is interpreted by Green as not falling within the scope of what is expected. And we see this in the doctor's question: *So, what part is important for such a drastic change?*

Garber's (1992) study indicates that the majority of transsexuals applying for reassignment are male. Most practitioners involved in sex-change programmes are males who often exhibit bias towards male patients and discourage women who enquire for treatment. These biases are reflected in the technology: for instance, the lack of significant advance on the construction of penises (or *phalloplasty*). According to Garber (1992) the amount of research funded and carried out in this direction makes sex changes for women less common and less clinically successful, despite the fact that the first total reconstruction of the penis was carried out in 1936. These gender biases and other reflections concerning the fact that transsexualism is (currently) a predominantly male phenomenon will be discussed further in later sections.

The rhetorics of GICs

> You are supposed to start your new life with an entirely new and unambiguously feminine name and forget the old one . . . you are supposed to have 'lived' and 'dressed' as a woman for three years . . . You're supposed to really believe you're a woman trapped in a man's body. (Vincent, 1993, p. 7)

Medical and legal discourses played an active part in the attribution of sex to ambiguous cases in the context of the eighteenth century (Foucault, 1979b, 1985). Nowadays gender identity programmes are active parts of these discourses. In order to go from one side of the sex-boundary to the other, candidates have to adjust their performance so as to fit into the psychiatric category of the opposite sex (Stone, 1991). This basic demand means that there is no possibility for ambiguity even during the hormonal treatment when both sexes' attributes are present. With regard to male-to-female transsexuals, Stone (1991, p. 286) states that they go 'from being unambiguous men, albeit unhappy men, to unambiguous women. There is no territory between'. Transsexuals are therefore also asked to erase a past body and sexual and social experiences which may 'interfere' with the adjustment to the other sex. These types of constraints include the requirement to dress and behave according to the stereotype of the gender they want to achieve physically for at least two years. In the passage below Dr Green explains to 'Todd' the rationale of this period known as the 'trial period'.

> *RG*: We want people who think they might want to have the surgery, which is irreversible, to first try on the real-life test, to experiment with what it's like on a day-to-day basis, to present oneself to the world as a woman. It takes practice in terms of use of cosmetics, dressing, walking, relating to people. It takes a lot of practice and time and trial. (Taken from Green, 1987, p. 130)

The important point here is that, in most cases, an individual's confusion of her/his sexual sense is presented as extremely distressing and damaging. The trial period thus reinforces a binary oppositional mode of gender identification. GICs demand purity and deny mixture (Stone, 1991).

The foundational discourses of GICs and their coordination of heterogeneous groups

Heterogeneous groups of human and non-human actors are coordinated in gender reassignment programmes. The different parts of the programmes work together to regulate the transgendered psyche. In particular, psychologists and counsellors become adjustors in order to control gender fluctuations and/or dissidence. For example, Stone relates how, in male-to-female transsexual communities, during the pre-operational phase nobody mentions practices such as 'wringing the turkey's neck' (or masturbation). This is because it questions the ideal shift from one sex to another and renders what is in between it as hidden or invisible (Stone, 1991, p. 289).

In the following we highlight the mutual, though asymmetrical, enrolment of clients, practitioners, institutions and, in more general terms, gender technologies that are used to perpetuate gender policies. We analyse these processes in both global and situated contexts. Borrowing some ideas from authors in the sociology of scientific knowledge and in particular the model of translation (Latour, 1986; Callon, 1991), the selection criteria and the trial period could be considered as a 'problematization moment' in which the dispersed parts involved in GICs are brought together into a shared space (gender reassignment programmes) and with a single purpose (to carry out the sex-change operation). These associations become possible by means of putting into circulation intermediaries which coordinate the many participants (Latour, 1986).

We now indicate how the logic of boundary objects, as framed by the model of translation, may also highlight tensions and dissidence within sex-change programmes. In doing so our claim is to explore additional ways of addressing our primary preoccupation in this book with recognizing and elaborating forms of resistance.

Boundary objects: shifting from within

Institutions and their policies do not exist as such: they are continually acted. A politically informed discursive approach helps us to analyse their everyday routines. ANT allows us to show that processes of standardization require constant work to reinforce the multiple associations which take place in local settings. Associations are established by means of boundary objects which are always open to interpretation. According to Star and Griesemer (1989), boundary objects are flexible enough to adapt to local needs and robust enough to be recognized and to survive across sites. This definition connects with the discourse analytical approach adopted in this chapter in which we identify and analyse practices whose dynamics are performed, maintained and renewed in local settings in a systematic, rather than random, way. Collective and organized readings of the ambiguities and the performative aspect of

Ángel Juan Gordo López

boundary objects may perform paradoxical and unintended effects and, among these, give rise to new possibilities of resistance. This generative aspect of interpretation can, for instance, be noted in the analysis of the dynamics of discussion groups (Gordo-López, 1995a; Gordo López and Georgaca, 1993). Voloshinov's (1973 [1929]) sociological analysis of language also regards the processes of evaluation as the generative aspect of meaning and social order. These evaluations are always the product of a collective configuration or of socially mediated (symbolic) interactions with linguistic, socio-technological fields of constraints (de Lauretis, 1989).

From a similar performative and local concern, authors such as Bowers and Middleton (1992) have pointed out the importance of interpretative work in understanding the flux of the organizations and how their information and patterns of coalition (structure) are performed by means of continuous interpretations in local settings. These interpretations entail a continuous adaptation and revitalization of multiplicity which prevents them from being assimilated by competing networks. This performative dimension of the standardization process is also noted by Star and Griesemer (1989, p. 408), who state that boundary objects are 'not engineered as such by any one individual or group, but rather emerged through the process of the work'. On the other hand, these interpretations are generative of new possibilities.

Returning to GICs, some of these interpretations prompt many predictable and unpredictable associations. For instance, some candidates work with feminist groups which train them in order to pass the selection interviews. Some of these groups focus on the study of the standards of the gender clinic at Charing Cross Hospital, London. Another association is that established between applicants and medical sources, as we have already illustrated in relation to the boundary object nature of Benjamin's (1966) book. Benjamin's (1966) book was used by different actors to achieve different discursive effects. But in so doing GICs' dynamics were not disrupted. Just the opposite: the degree of coordination between the different parts was 'highly' satisfactory.

At this point, several key aspects should be noted regarding the dynamics of GICs and their virtual, discursive and material technologies of gender. First, GICs are rigid networks whose coordination is achieved by means of flexible boundary objects. GICs prescribe transsexuals' performance, wishes and identities by speaking on behalf of the candidates (or 'translate'[1] them). Second, rigid networks can be assimilated by more heterogeneous and informal networks related to them, such as the network created between candidates and feminist support groups. Third, by means of aligning with feminist support groups, transsexuals introduce multiplicity into the programmes of GICs. In this process they learn how to perform rhetorical identities in order to proceed through the programme, rather than merely adapt to stereotyped gender views. Thus they create different networks and identities that can 'move about the network[s]'.[2] Fourth, and finally, these new associations allow the transsexual multiple positions from which she/he can 'perform' (in the theatrical sense) identities in GICs, rather than 'acquire' them before disappearing into the heterosexual population. It is the difference between (dramaturgical) *performing* and (the developmental psychological notion of) *acquiring* that confers political relevance to the terminological distinction between 'sex change' and 'gender reassignment'.

Contributing to already existing counter-discourses: conferring voice to silenced locations

> Boundaries shift from within; boundaries are very tricky. What boundaries provisionally contain remains generative, productive of meaning and bodies. Siting (sighting) boundaries is a risky practice. (Haraway, 1991, p. 201)

We now highlight the value of making visible *high risk zones* to recover for analysis the doubts or tensions involved in the 'game' of 'passing'. Through this we contribute to the project of cultural politics of gender ambiguity and the recent work in queer theory of describing 'those possibilities that already exist, but which exist within cultural domains designated as culturally unintelligible and impossible' (Butler, 1990b, pp. 148–9).

Examples of zones of high risk

Star (1991) comments on the experience of one of her students (Jan) working in Silicon Valley, who decided to take up health insurance for the expensive process of transsexual surgery. During the trial period Jan/Janice started dressing in a gender-neutral way and came to enjoy the experience so much that s/he doubted if s/he wanted to go ahead with the surgery:

> It's like being in a very high tension zone, as if something's about to explode . . . People can't handle me this way – they want me to be one thing or another. But it's also really great, I'm learning so much about what it means to be neither one nor the other. (Jan, quoted in Star, 1991, p. 45)

Though Janice eventually completed the last phases of the change of sex, she was able to benefit from those 'zones of high tensions'. Another example of high tension worth indicating is the *Barrymore* programme on Granada (shown Saturday, 12 February 1994) broadcast at peak time for a British audience (7.30 pm). In this programme there was an interview with a post-transsexual and a pre-transsexual who, like Janice, did not want to complete the last phase of her/his change. While this person was lying on the couch (that is, they were treating her as a psychiatric subject in need of mental health services) the audience was asked if they found this middle position between sexes/genders offensive. In contrast to the policies of GICs and other (representations of) mass-media opinion, *Barrymore*'s audience professed not to find this person's ambiguous position offensive.

Transhomosexuality and the denial of a postmodern gender/sexual location

As Tully (1992) indicates, the term 'transhomosexuality' was coined by the psychiatrist and author Clare in 1984 to refer to those people who want to become a member of the opposite sex in order to have homosexual relationships. Transhomosexuals are often categorized as a subcategory of transsexuals by psychiatrists and the rhetorics of GICs. The following extract presents a male diagnosed as transhomosexual speaking about some of his/her sexual ambiguities. Given the pathologization of so-called transhomosexuality, it is worth reflecting on whether this differs from heterosexual relationships:

> When I am highly sexually aroused I will escape entirely from my fantasies of the female role. After ejaculation everything goes back to normal and the two roles coexist . . . Everything the 'he part' wants to do is different to the 'she part'. If 'he' does the washing up, this challenges the 'she part' . . . When I am less aroused and my current girlfriend comes on top of me I think of her penetrating me. (Taken from Tully, 1992, p. 141)

Nevertheless, these fluctuations are considered by GICs as indicative of not having reached a final transsexual status. However, we consider them as fluctuations which manifest continuous shifts or positions in between, as the following extract illustrates:

> I feel very much neuter between what a man and a woman is. My identity should be a woman's but really I am in a no-woman's land. People don't see me the way I see women . . . I have wondered if I can be happy to accept my transsexualism and not live as a woman. There is conflict between my male erections and need for orgasms, and my physical libidinal desires as a female. (Male-to-female, taken from Tully, 1992, p. 178)

It is relevant that most of the biomedical research on transsexualism and the mass media do not mention the existence of transhomosexuals. Is this undocumented aspect of transhomosexuality related to the policies of GICs where the project of gender reassignment makes invisible dissonant gender/sex possibilities? Or is it a contributor, and index of, the growth of the surgical industry? The transhomosexual position requires a work of 'location' (Probyn, 1990) within GICs. Transhomosexuals are displaced through this process of fixation in relation to an already structured web of practices determined by a medical psychiatric discourse, to a subcategory of transsexualism. This has to be overcome in order to be eligible for sex-change operations. By attending to these processes of 'positionality' (Burman, 1994b) we could explore the textual production of (transsexuals') identities and, doing so, to contribute to dis/locating the institutional boundaries of GICs. For example, it is possible that transsexuals do not easily adjust to the slogans floating in GICs: 'I am trapped in the wrong body' and 'I want to change sex to become a normal citizen'. It might also be the case that the policies of GICs do not allow the possibility of passing from one 'aberrant' position ('I want to change sex') to another (to become homosexual/lesbian). These regulatory practices inform the structure of GICs which define the array of possible eligible positions while excluding other possibilities.

Opening up doubts and contradictions in medical and legal discourse

There are continuous difficulties in the diagnoses of transsexualism and disagreements within the medical practices about the origins of these 'abnormal' gender positions. There is no research which guarantees a biological structure accounting for gender identity and its many manifestations. For instance, an article (Lonsdale, 1993, p. 25) entitled 'When sex-change is a mistake' stresses the negative aspect, reporting a psychiatrist talking about Sandra, a postoperational transsexual, who is suffering in her current condition and who 'was in reality a gay man trying to deny her homosexuality'. Using the pronoun 'her' qualifying 'a gay man' inadvertently works to challenge the supposedly unitary nature of sexual identities at the moment of asserting it.

The bedrock of research on transsexualism is the account of its aetiology. According to Stoller (1975), the origins of transsexual gender dysphoria are to be found in the Oedipal stage of psychosexual development. The mother is often depicted as the responsible agent (see Green, 1987, for a discussion of how 'Todd's' mother is presented as the origins of her son's 'deviation'). However, later studies have not found any link between family relationship and transsexuality (Lothstein, 1983). Moreover, sex-reassignment programmes have drawn on cognitive developmental psychology (e.g. Kohlberg, 1969) which presumes that gender identity is formed in the early years, being stabilized afterwards. This has not been ratified by later research (Tully, 1992).

Despite the lack of any medical survey or evidence to support the argument that transsexual candidates are more likely to suffer psychological breakdowns or crises than any others, transsexuals are often pathologized. This is illustrated by a psychiatrist's comments regarding her work in a GIC: 'You have to remember that people who believe they are transsexuals are often in a terrible state, depressed, worried' (reported by Lonsdale, 1993, p. 25). Furthermore, gender reassignments of the British NHS do not correspond with legal practices. The birth certificate remains as the proof of a person's sex (Davies, 1990, p. 17; Vincent, 1993, p. 7). This entails the lack of legal recognition of the transsexual's new sex. This is another example of the hierarchical structure of these types of practices. A legal discourse is fixed to a biological discourse, even though the biological shape can be changed by cultural choice, technological support and institutionalized practices. These tensions were made explicit in the case taken up by Caroline Cossey who challenged British law to recognize her as a woman after her sex-change operation. Although the European Court of Human Rights criticized the failure of English law to recognize marriages between transsexuals, Caroline could not mobilize enough support to change the sex on her birth certificate (Davies, 1990, p. 17).

Invasion across gender empires: moral gender tales?

Gender biases can be noticed in recent British mass media. Most newspaper articles mention that transsexualism is a male phenomenon (male-to-female transsexual). For instance Vincent (1993, p. 4) in the article 'Lost Boys' published in *The Guardian* states that

> transsexualism is a predominantly male phenomenon and it prolifer- ates at an alarming rate as an example of the extraordinary things men will do to one another when they have the power, the techno- logy and the licence to practise them.

It is significant that only one of the articles I came across during the course of my doctoral research this chapter draws on presents the case of a 'female-to- male transsexual'. This article by Udall (1994) was published in the British tabloid newspaper *The People* (16 January). This example enables us to visu- alize associations between the androcentric tradition in transsexualism and the sensationalist way (commodity-like – Irigaray, 1985) in which this female-to- male transsexual example is presented to public opinion. In some newspaper tabloids the sensationalist style is evident in massage services and sexual appearance transformation shop advertisements (as we discuss below), as well as female pornography. In contrast, most of the articles published about transsexualism in 'quality' papers such as *The Guardian*, *The Observer* and *The Independent* mainly addressed different aspects and discourses concerning male-to-female transsexuals.

Thus female-to-male sex exchanges are still news; its 'freakish' monstros- ity and novelty amuse and/or disturb public opinion. It participates of the carnivalesque as the 'unruly' *women* which both invites and indulges desires for morbidity and scandal in the dominant gendered psyche (Chapter 9). Its counterpart, male-to-female transsexuals, are no longer profitable. But it has become part of our everyday news or, paraphrasing Barthes (1977, p. 165), a reflection of the natural, a matter of course, the norm, the *doxa*. This logic of morbidity and gender-biased naturalizing effects, which seems to motivate market policies as well as directing some readings, has been discussed in terms of 'invasion' and 'envy' by some feminist authors.

Shapiro (1991) comments on some sociological studies on transsexuals carried out by Kando (1973) which show the high degree of gender conservatism found among the transsexual community: 'Unlike various liberated groups, transsexuals are reactionary, moving back toward the core-culture rather than away from it' (Kando 1973, p. 145; quoted in Shapiro, 1991, p. 255). The conservative attitude is not the only reason why some women and some feminist scholars find transsexuals disturbing. According to these views, male-to-female transsexuals are men who acquire robotically stereotyped gender manners, shapes, clothes, cosmetics and, indeed, womanhood, visualized/made from/by the male perspective. This reading of transsexuality raises many hostilities and great indignation. For instance, in the different newspaper articles analysed there was a common account that coincides with Kando's results: 'Male-to-female transsexuals tested higher in femininity than women' (Shapiro, 1991, p. 253).

Raymond's (1979) book *The Transsexual Empire: The Making of the She-Male* develops one of the most influential feminist critiques of transsexualism. As Shapiro indicates, Raymond thinks of transsexuals as intruders into women's worlds who want to divide and control women once again by adopting female forms. Some of Raymond's views about male-to-female are as follows: 'All transsexuals rape women's bodies by reducing the female form to an artifact, appropriating this body for themselves . . . Rape, athough it is usually done by force, can also be accomplished by deception' (Raymond, 1979; quoted in Stone, 1991, p. 283). Raymond's arguments can be placed within a Western feminist politics that relies on the notion of 'consciousness raising' or 'awareness' predicated on the production (or exploration) of identity. These politics are also built on definitions of 'womanhood based on historical/biographical experience and one defined biologically in terms of sex' (Shapiro, 1991, p. 259). Thus Raymond's suspicion of transsexuals resembles the current suspicions of some feminist politics of identities and their critique of the postmodernist overvaluation of the 'feminine' narrative. Authors such as Brodribb (1992) and Jackson (1992) comment on the feminization (or 'transsexualization') of postmodernist thought (and the *matrix* and cyborg bodies within it – Wolmark, 1995), arguing that the referents for the postmodern feminist are none other than great male master theorists such as Lacan, Derrida, Foucault, Deleuze and Lyotard. For these feminist scholars, postmodernist feminist endeavours may risk the 'body' erasing the marginal position of women and the discourses which struggle against the material and social conditions of gender asymmetries.

However, from a discursive perspective, the notion of boundary objects helps us to think of the transsexual body in the wider context of the discourses and institutions which reshape it as part of its historical/biographical experience. It also helps us to understand its production within situated practices in interaction with material and symbolic elements. Boundary objects, in a similar way to some performative understandings of gender (Butler, 1990b), call for a situatedness and coordination of the multiple body of knowledges and technologies to make sense of the local (Haraway, 1991). This focus on the local does not imply that boundary objects do not consider wider sexual and gender policies, of which GICs are only a fragment.

In a similar vein, Stone refers to Raymond's notion of invasion and her ideas about the body, gender and politics as being about 'morality tales and origin myths, about telling the "truth" of gender' (Stone, 1991, p. 284). Raymond's critique seems to forget that transsexuals are effects of wider 'gender factories' and possible emplacements for sexual dissidence (Dollimore, 1991) and trans-citizenship (Evans, 1993). I consider it more politically effective to investigate the interplays between constraints and empowerment rather than criticizing (thereby fixing them) as standardized products available from the gender empire and/or factory. Or in other words: how many empires would we need to locate anger, envy and hate against diffuse gendered/sexual referents? As Stone (1991) indicates, the story is about the inscriptions and reading practices of late capitalism. The discursive reformulation of boundary objects framed here and their resemblance with power flux, as we shall exemplify below, enable us to move from local settings and everyday practice to wider social gender/sexuality policies and back again to local fields. It also challenges social constructionist approaches in psychology, for example via cyberpsychology (Burman *et al.*, 1995; Gordo López, 1995b), to develop perspectives in which knowledge and technologies are not separate from the context that surrounds them, but combine to include the flux of information, the human body and its sexual/gender performances.

New gender and sexual possibilities in the late capitalist market: 'travesti' boys from Brazil and four cross-dressing hours to discover the true inner self

A high price for the challenge of nature/social standards: 'Boys from Brazil'

The term *travesti* does not exist in the English language. The closest term is 'transvestite' which refers to heterosexual men who like to wear women's clothes or dress in a cross-gendered way. Travesti is used to designate a man who grows breasts with the help of hormones and in many cases injects silicone into muscle tissue to produce a feminine form, but the penis is not removed as in a full transsexual operation. In a TV documentary programme screened on

British TV about Brazilian 'travestis', they were identified as: 'people who choose to be both male and female. Hormone treatment and silicon implants give them women's bodies but they still have male genitalia. They are called "travestis". There is no word for them yet in English' (*Boys from Brazil*, BBC2, UK, May 1993).

In contrast to transsexuals, these 'Boys from Brazil' obtain hormone treatment and plastic surgery by unofficial practitioners and private clinics. They inject themselves or get non-professionals to inject industrial silicon into their hips and as a result they often suffer from fatal infections. This happened to Luciana whose hips became saggy and infected. Luciana says to the doctor: 'I'll get to Italy as soon as I'm better. I'll have to have plastic surgery once the silicon has been removed. As you remove the silicon the skin becomes saggy. So I'll need to have plastic surgery, creams, exercises, things like that. Then I'll be a new woman with a dick! [laughing] ahy!' (*Boys from Brazil*, BBC2, UK, May 93). Travestis, therefore, negotiate ambiguous positions by means of unofficial practices. As Luciana states, 'a travesti is neither man nor woman. Everyone can tell what we are. But some, as you can see, are very feminine.'

Nevertheless, it is important to recall the social context from which people such as these 'Boys from Brazil' emerge: they maintain themselves by prostitution and derive from the deprived social classes of the already exoticized and eroticized 'Third World' countries. These marginal positions (in recent mass-media referred to as 'the third sex' – e.g. Howarth's article about 'Miss Dandys' in Japan, in *Marie Claire*, June 1994) add a new inflection to the term 'boundary object' as commodity form and relation. As a male Italian client states in this TV programme to account for his sexual preference for these 'Boys from Brazil':

> It's a new phenomenon and like new phenomena especially those relating to sex we are very responsive to them. They come from South America and poorer Third World countries. We're attracted to them. The look of their faces, the shape of their eyes and many other things. It's something exotic and deeply perverted. (*Boys from Brazil*, BBC2, UK, May 1993)

The condition of 'Boys from Brazil', therefore, emerges from a textuality distinct from the one maintained by GICs. Their location may be understood from below, from the position of the marginal and deprived. This can some-times challenge established sexual orders in their regulated moves across multiple memberships and countries and private cosmetic surgeries, beyond where money goes and beyond 'trial' periods of gender change. In their economic transactions across dominant understandings of sexual borderlands, 'Boys from Brazil' may question the heterosexuality of the Italian clients that are eventually positioned in a 'hetero'-sexual relationship in the sense of diffuse identification with the object of their desire. It is also worth noticing at this point that the accounts of these 'Boys from Brazil' are different from those accounts of candidates for sex-change operations in Western GICs. Travestis present themselves as active agencies, sometimes involved in magic and religious rituals, who are able to confront nature and/or God's willingness. The following extracts exemplify Samira's (formerly Bobby Fontana) challenge of Nature and God's fate (numbers in brackets indicate pauses in seconds):

Samira: If I were to be born again. God would decide my destiny. I'd accept the gender He bestowed upon me. I didn't accept it this time, because I was born with both sexes [³ she says *duo problemas*]. I think God is a little to blame. He should have clearly defined my gender. I would have accepted whatever I was born with. But this way I've had to define it myself. Because the side I feel most at ease with is my feminine side . . . My entity is Pomba-Gira, Lucifer's wife. Many people have a spirit which is half man, half woman. They will choose a body which is both man and woman. That is why this spirit felt at home in my body . . .

Interviewer: What happened to Bobby Fontana?

Samira: Basically, I killed him. [1.5] Because that wasn't Bobby Fontana's true identity. His true identity is the one I have now and that has been assumed for a long time now. (*Boys from Brazil*, BBC2, UK, May 1993)

Samira positions herself beyond nature and moral restrictions. She, as an emerging effect of wider socio-technological conditions, is able to mobilize positions from which to decide about his/her sexual aesthetics, fate or gender beliefs. Adopting Foucault's (1979b) terms, this ethical axis entails a process of subjectification in which enjoyment and politics intermingle in a context of prostitution, body danger, suffering and Nietzschean 'laughter': 'G: It's as if we're from another planet. We should all be called 'Suffering' (*sufridos*) because we all suffer so much! [laughter]' (*Boys from Brazil*, BBC2, UK, May 1993)

Thus travestis' locations can be considered as a culturally unintelligible domain (Butler, 1990b) in which agency emerges from constraints and epistemic violence (Spivak, 1988, 1989; Bourdieu and Wacquant, 1992); a domain in which the ethical, the political, the subjective and the marginal coexist in local settings and across several countries and (sexual) market economies. These positions are not recognized by specialized institutions like GICs. But both sets of institutions may also be situated in the political unconscious of our late capitalism and its ever more flexible process of accumulation.

The political unconscious and 'new exciting transvestite changeaways'

As an example of the logic of accumulation and the local and malleable aspect of postmodern identities we now discuss new types of advertisements in English tabloid newspapers. The adverts below (Figures 10.1 and 10.2) have regularly appeared from late 1993 in *The People* (e.g. 16 January 1994) and *The Mirror* (e.g. 7 November 1993).

As Figure 10.3 illustrates, such advertisements appear in the context of 'Sexy Rubber Panties', 'Ladies Change Your Man ['s underwear]', 'Adult XXX films' (*The People*, 16 January 1994). It is now possible to enjoy a sex-boundary transgression for a few hours at a reasonable price. Are these adverts related to the wider practices of boundaries objects? Would this postmodernist feature of play with sex/gender ambiguity stop people from waiting to change sex? They can indulge their fantasy and still maintain 'family values'.

These are examples of the way a free-floating postmodernist logic coexists with the flexible specialization of late capitalist production. They can also be thought of as part of a more global network of sex/gender subjectivities and identities in which GICs are active sites. The 'new exciting transvestite changeaways' offer the discovery of the 'true inner self' in the period of (only) four hours (see Figure 10.1). This is possible by means of a vast range of

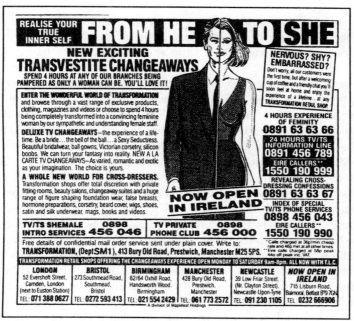

Figure 10.1 'Realise Your True Inner Self: From He to She' (*The Mirror, 7 November 1993*)

Ángel Juan Gordo López

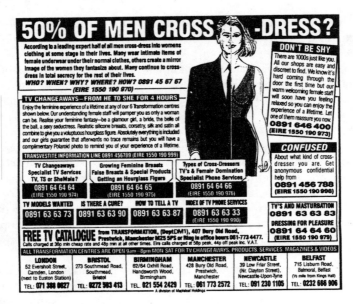

Figure 10.2 '50% of Men Cross-Dress?' (*The People, 16 January 1994*)

artefacts and prostheses that reshape the malleable physical body. As it appears in the advert, some of those are: 'false breasts, hormone preparations, corsetry, beard covers, wigs, shoes, satin and silk underwear, mags, books and videos'.

The society of the media and spectacle, or of multinational capitalism, endorses the mutability of the body (mostly women's bodies – Smith, 1990). However this mutability may be also understood as a way to erase confusion for a few hours: managing variety but prolonging the sexual *status quo*. In this, many sexual agencies and locations are produced within our specialized late capitalism production: doing business with sexually 'aberrant' positions while accounting for variability. As in Marcuse's (1968) notion of 'repressive tolerance', this controls the margins of variation or 'sex transformation'.

Another example of how technological advances and aesthetics of consumption have erupted into the postmodern landscape of virtual transformations includes the ways virtual reality affords new arenas of enterprise to owners of chains of transformation sex-shops. At the latest International Conference on Virtual Reality some transformation shop owners persistently asked for the price of high-end VR systems, foreseeing the new possibilities for customers in 'virtual cross-dressing' environments (Macauley and Gordo López, 1995).

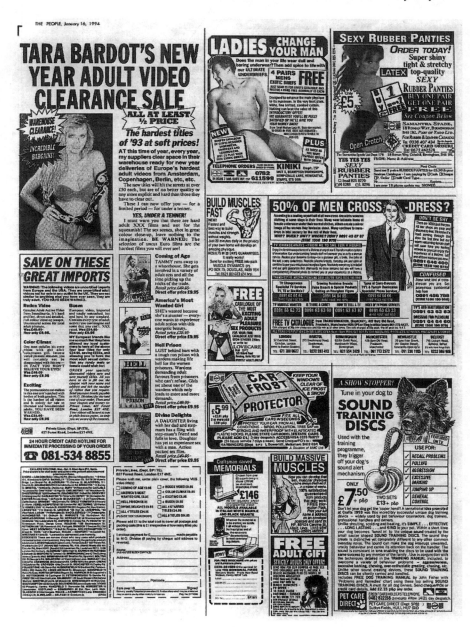

Figure 10.3 Context of advertising of Cross-Dressing Shops (*The People, 16 January 1994*)

Ángel Juan Gordo López

From regulation to resistance

The notion of boundary objects has been put forward to develop a critical analysis of the way social dynamics, including sex/gender policies, regulate economies of the body and its pleasures. GICs and their medical and psychological discourses are simply one fragment of these dynamics. This chapter has also illustrated how groups of practitioners are coordinated by boundary objects, constructing their patients as transsexuals. Transsexualism in these clinics has been depicted as a boundary object which serves to produce, prolong and maintain binary sexual and gender divisions. We have also illustrated the way these boundary objects are sensitive to wider social practices such as the ones expressed/maintained by articles, advertisements and documentaries in the British mass media. This confers on the analysis a wider social dimension which also informs the commodity and relational aspect of the term 'boundary object'. And it is the paradoxical relational aspects of it as commodity which enables us to move from local settings and everyday practices to wider social gender/sexuality policies and back again to local fields of constraints in order to articulate and sight new and/or already existing strategies for resistance.

Regulations and/or technical devices are open to interpretation and multiple uses. Even surgical technologies have a discursive genealogy (as we have seen in the example of female-to-male transsexuals). As numerous feminists have documented, artefacts do have both gender and politics (Berg and Lie, 1993; Cockburn and Fürst-Dili, 1994). As Balka (1993, p. 11) notes, 'technological products both bear the imprint of their social context, and themselves reinforce [and/or subvert] that social context'. Surgical advances, legal and medical discourse as well as institutions afford transgressive and challenging interpretation within their regulatory fields of constraints. Gender technologies and relations are, like the sexual body, both material and discursive. It is important to emphasize this in order to widen and support the range of available points of resistance.

Currently, in relation to these perspectives, Foucault's writings are, at best, elusive. So are most discursive approaches within social psychology. Although most of these approaches have begun to be recognized (and often translated into recuperable forms) in our institutions, they do not highlight the alternative ways of conceptualizing resistance in institutional settings where the discipline of psychology is used in oppressive ways including our educational establishments (Gordo López and Linaza, 1996). As Ibáñez (1995) argues, changes happen with the articulation of new practices within psychology. We need politically committed architects (and technicians) of resistance. This chapter, and in general this book, has aimed to stimulate that sort of readings and practices. Some of us have found feminists' work such as Butler's (1990b) extremely helpful (see Chapters 6, 8 and 9) when highlighting 'culturally unintelligible and impossible domains' in order to bring up tensions ('dissonance') in the politics of location (Spivak, 1988; Probyn, 1990; Bondi, 1993).

Nevertheless, these sorts of projects need more specific analysis which includes, for instance, the technologies of gender in their multiple 'material-discursive' aspects. Otherwise our politics will ignore the mediational and discursive character of these technologies (Gordo López, 1995a).

Furthermore, it is not enough to identify practices which regulate the body and gender. Coalitions and alternative alliances with people who participate in these practices should be strengthened. A high degree of coordination is needed to organize and mobilize those 'cultural unintelligible categories' such as those people who want to retain their ambiguous sexual/gender identities within gender-reassignment programmes. To legitimize these sort of locations we need stronger networks and relational analytical devices to mediate and free-associate in more efficient ways. As committed people (and psychologists), we should find alternative boundary objects or develop alternative interpretations of already existing ones. These including action-oriented networks against oppressive psychological uses such as the organization Psychology Politics Resistance (Reicher and Parker, 1993) to support, for instance, those feminist groups which train transsexuals to perform, rather than acquire, identities. And for this we also need boundary objects such as computer-mediated databases in order to coordinate, organize and distribute individual resources from different sites including psychologists' institutional settings and technologies (*PPR Newsletter #1*, Autumn, 1994). In short, discursive-analytical work concerned with more efficient and wider paths of resistance should take seriously the ways socio-technological dynamics are undetachable from the origins and functioning of the psychological *apparatus* (or 'psy-techno-complexes', Gordo López, 1995a).

Acknowledgments

I am grateful to Owens Heathcote, Julia Varela, Pep García-Borés and the co-authors of this book for their comments and discussion on earlier versions of the paper. Without Erica Burman's and Ian Parker's intellectual and personal support this work, as well as other parts of my thesis research, would not have been possible.

Notes

1 ANT describes the dynamics of associations with the aid of the linguistic metaphor of 'translation'. The term 'translation' implies transformation. Translation is also akin to persuasion and/or cooperation: 'One actant manages to persuade others to fall into line, it thereby increases its strengths and becomes stronger than those it aligned and convinced' (Latour, 1988, p. 172). Law (1992) contemplates translations as a social process which generates 'ordering effects' such as agents, institutions and organizations.

2 To take a parallel example for this third point, Singleton and Michael (1993) analyse the part played by the general practitioners in the cervical screening programme (CSP) in the UK. The GPs are depicted as the centralizing actor (or boundary object) for the success of CSP. However, Singleton and Michael stress that the multiplicity introjected in the network (laboratory workers, women recipients, cervical cells, cervical cancer, etc.) was based on the ambivalence adopted by GPs towards the CSP. In particular the GPs' multiple identities, rather than their simplification, determined the degree in which GPs enrolled women to pass the tests.
3 This includes my translation of parts of the conversations in Portuguese omitted by the translation into English subtitle.

Postscripts

In this section we comment on issues emerging from the themes and process of this book. As a co-written piece, like this co-authored book, we do not aim to try and tidy up or summarize the differences and tensions between the chapters that comprise this volume. Rather, here we attempt to open them up and elaborate what they and the critical projects described in the previous chapters mean for turning psychology's regulation into resistance. So in these postscripts we want to draw attention to the disagreements and shifts of perspective which have characterized the elaboration of this book. In broader terms, we see these as reflections of tensions in discursive analytical research, at least in the context of our work around the Discourse Unit at the Manchester Metropolitan University. As Parker (1995, p. 1) indicates, 'the multiplicity of meaning in a discourse calls for a multiplicity of vantage points and theoretical frameworks, and a multiplicity of subject positions'. The tensions and intersections in the book and the resource for these postscripts reproduce wider political and theoretical debates in the social sciences. We identify key tensions around the issues of regulation and resistance, modernity and postmodernity, relativism and materiality, processes and effects and the textual and technophilic body. Finally, we consider the coalitions (as opposed to stable alliances) that include the one which formed the locus for this book and end with some comments on global identities and local pleasures.

Regulation and resistance

In this book we have been concerned with a range of practices which we have identified in different ways as either regulatory or as resources for resistance. Nevertheless, despite the coherence of project, differing conceptions of regulation and resistance are elaborated within different chapters, in part as a response to the specific arenas of practice being addressed, but also as a reflection of differences in theoretico-political orientations between us. A modernist reading of regulation and resistance would see these as opposites, as opposed to their infinitely complex permutations according to postmodernists and Foucauldians (see later). Thus in discussion with each other and over time we were sometimes able to distinguish regulation from resistance for pragmatic purposes and in relation to individuals and institutions; at others, we saw the intersections between power and knowledge as so bound together and unpredictable that they shaded into each other. Still, our concern has been with how these dynamics of power/knowledge are invested in flesh, individuals and institutions.

Despite our concern to engage in reflective and grounded critique, we have been aware of how we could not avoid sometimes reifying these concepts. This was reflected in bizarrely clear ways within the discussions we had over whether a particular chapter should be put in the 'regulation' or 'resistance' sections of the book. Towards the end, we began to doubt how much it mattered how we drew up the book 'sections' because the chapters could be read in different ways (as either more focused on resistance or regulation). Further, despite attempting to be more sophisticated than this, we generally found ourselves drawing up an opposition between the resisting subject fighting an oppressive and regulatory 'Goliath' of psychology. Yet ultimately the real world, as Foucault recognized, is more complex than our concepts can convey. The boundary between regulation and resistance is in constant flux and depends where one is positioned within the social matrix. There are also times when, as we have seen, aspects of psychological regulation, such as self-help manuals, are helpful. Nor would we want to suggest that some forms of self-regulation are not necessary or desirable.

In many ways, our struggle to offer an account of the complex interactions between subjects interpellated by familial, legal, educational, therapeutic, sexual and comic discourses is doomed to be reductive. The process of writing inevitably reproduces, mediates and transforms these discourses. As such, *Psychology Discourse Practice* is itself both a regulatory and resistant text. It has been our primary aim to tread a delicate path between telling a story about a range of practices and the multiple ways these practices position people and also telling a coherent story about inequality and oppression. But in doing the latter, we contribute to the creation of a new 'textualizing' discourse which produces a new set of effects and positions. We cannot control or predict the effects of this book on you as reader, student, practitioner, client or researcher. Ultimately, in this set of postscripts, we do not wish to resolve all the loose theoretical ends of the multifarious stories we have told. Rather, we wish merely to note their presence and some of the dilemmas and intrinsic paradoxes with which we all, as critical researchers, struggle.

Power

Power has been a central theme throughout this book. As authors, we shared a core concern with the power that psychological discourses have in (and increasingly beyond) contemporary Western culture. In a multitude of ways, each chapter is involved in mapping the power of psychological discourses in particular locations and in relation to the resistances and negotiations of power that people can and do provide. While in some chapters the focus is more on potential positions of resistance (e.g. Chapters 6, 7 and 8), in others (e.g. Chapters 2 and 3) it is on actual positions that we illustrate. We have tried to show how forces of power and resistance are movements in continual struggle which we sometimes prise apart in order to examine them politically and theoretically.

Beyond this, there are differences in the precise models of power that the authors of different chapters draw on. While all are informed by post-structuralist ideas, further subdivisions might distinguish those who would primarily identify themselves with Marxist or feminist-inspired readings of post-structuralism and those more informed by more recent work associated with queer theory. Furthermore, some chapters make the issue of conceptualizing power an explicit theme (e.g. Chapters 3, 6 and 8), while for others it is its operation at specific points that is of concern, or particular aspects of its operation (such as through particular psychological divisions and classifications).

Issues of power are intimately bound up with the presentation of expertise. As authors we are each placed in particular ways as regards our 'expertise'; as practitioners (clinical psychologists, educational psychologists, therapists, as researchers in 'the field', etc.). However, although in writing these chapters we are also each claiming the position of academic practitioner because we are all authors in the present text and hence positioned as experts through conventional networks of meanings.

Related to this is the issue of reflexivity. Taking up positions of authorship in the production of this text renders us powerful. Inevitably, we replicate the standard positions of the author having voice and the lack of voice for readers of the text, which has traditionally implied a passive reception on the part of the reader. After considerable discussion, we chose to allow authors of individual chapters to determine the extent to which they would place themselves explicitly in their writing, to reflect on their positions (either in relation to their topic or their text), or to adopt dominant academic conventions such as the impersonal tone and third-person style of writing. We decided to adopt more or less reflexive positions according to the focus of our chapters, our particular relation to the material and our belief in the relevance and significance of authorial positioning within the chapter.

Tensions and intersections

A major tension related to current debates about whether or not losing identities implies losing claims to political agendas and notions of 'the real'. So there are moments in this book where we recognize that the fluidity of identities may entail a denial of both material reality and the dynamics of oppression. On other occasions we find it helpful to draw on the politics associated with postmodern notions rather than invoking secure identity or even subjectivity (Butler, 1992). In this way and attending to the specificity of

our particular topics of study, we have also thrown some of the presuppositions of identity politics into question by highlighting the relational basis of
identification (Burman, 1994b, p. 173). A third position also reflected in our
analyses is the development of useful encounters between the (feminist) politics of identities and postmodernist relational views (such as the logics of
locations: Spivak, 1989; Probyn, 1990; Bondi, 1993).

From often opposed, but collectively formed, positions, our accounts of
the dynamics of regulation and resistance have been placed in the high-risk
zones emerging from the interplay between modernity (e.g. humanism, Marxism, social constructionism, feminist politics of identities) and postmodernity
(relational and networking thinking, queer and performative understandings
of gender, agency and the body). These border zone tensions have been useful
and translatable into other politicized uses which include impurities, paradoxes and contradictions both within each chapter and between the different
chapters. Some of these post/modern tensions and stories that structured our
discussions can be exemplified as follows:

> *First Story*: Postmodernist approaches are coined by the mobile and
> educated middle class in late capitalism in which specialization and
> interdisciplinarity are both necessary qualities.

> *Second Story*: Right but erm, different subject positions are consti-
> tuted by different sets of practices and experiences which we cannot
> gather together under a common identity or political agendas.

> *First Story*: Multiplicity and all that postmodernist stuff [laughter]
> doesn't offer a well-developed analysis of the way local constraints
> may both regulate and empower individuals in concrete practices and
> this is a key aspect of this book.

> *Third Story*: Yeah. Right. No, everything is mobile. There is a need in
> concrete cases to keep sight of. Theorize material or extra-discursive
> practices.

> *Fourth Story*: It might be the case that material practices appear as if
> they were global immutable facts. It might also be the case that the
> naturalizing processes we are trying to identify.

> *Third Story*: Even if these material practices fall outside the discur-
> sive webs?

> *Fourth Story*: Hmmmm. Well. Erm, we also intend to situate and
> identify the continuous work of location. Who it interrelates with and
> how this produces conflict. Shifts and mutatations without neces-
> sarily subscribing our analyses to relativistic readings of discourse.

> *Dialogical We*: Right. The point here seems to be how we retain a
> realist suspicion of the social constructionist work in the ways we also

address different gradients of materiality of those extra-(and/or)-discursive practices.

Authors' shifts between these stories partly indicate the complexities of this co-authored 'we' and their disparate engagements. These also reflect some of the different social backgrounds, distinct class/gender consciousnesses and strategies of approaching the means of resistance according to our many arenas of study.

Materiality in the psy-complex: processes/effects

This book presents tensions between discursive effects and the construction and dislocation of the processes which support them. As with social constructionist work, the different perspectives in this book also face the problems of idealizing/abstracting rather than embodying those discursive effects. A primary preoccupation in this book has been attending to ways of elaborating resistance. In order to challenge oppressive and naturalizing practices our analyses have been interpellated by different gradients of discursive effects/processes, local/global perspectives, relativism/realisms and other axes of de/construction. According to different positions in these axes, the analytical and political tensions in this book include the following. We identify these practices' local constitution in broader institutional levels. We attend to processes and the effects that subordinate and pathologize deviations from the standards that they manufacture. We examine the ways they are reproduced across multiple sites. Our de/constructive work gains richness and strength from its analytical complexity and contradictions.

Moreover, another set of discrepancies unfold from the wide set of understandings of discourses and their associated uses. Some of these have highlighted aspects and forms of subjectivity aiming to challenge the assumptions that have structured the nets of psychology (its networks of meaning and corresponding enclosures of subjectivity). Our analyses are mainly concerned with the administration practices and oppressive effects of these psychological nets. Other analyses in this book have emphasized the technologies of (psycho and sexual) regulation in institutional contexts. We have conceived of these technologies as material, relational and discursive. Our positions here therefore draw on, but significantly develop, previous discursive-analytical and genealogical work in psychology which accords technologies the status of conceptual regimes (e.g. Rose, 1985, 1989). One theoretical claim arising from our work in this book is that such a perspective frequently fails to comprehend the different degrees of materiality of discourse.

These new types of analyses in psychology bring artefacts into agency and socialize technologies into discursive frames. This may be a way forward to 'expand the real' and develop notions of discourse which embrace relationships between physical organisms and artefacts, bodies and discourses.

Without such approaches we can only get a partial (and perhaps overly deterministic) view of discursive effects, which misconsider their processes of regulation. These considerations may take the form of adding politics to traditional ethnographic studies, or developing actor-network approaches in the discipline of the sociology of scientific knowledge. By adding materiality to the discursive construction of psychological practices, it may be possible to ward off relativist readings of discourses as merely social constructions floating free of material practices.

Textuality and technology

Throughout the production of this book we differed in our perspectives on technology. We have moved between a view of technologies as static products and as part of the processes and effects of the (psychological) nets where they are built and applied. Such readings prompted tensions and disagreements among our co-authored 'we' and reflect Marxist and feminist qualms about technology which have often equated technological advances with new forms of control. But from other readings and theoretical resources (see Chapter 1), we have also argued that organizational boundaries and their technologies do not exist as such: they are continually performed and maintained. From these perspectives power and its technologies are not capacities with pre-given designs and effects, but groups, actions and material agents mobilized and exercised *in situ*. If technologies (of power, gender, 'race', pathologization, education and mothering) are associated with (patriarchal) ruling practices and if these forms are groups of actions rather than capacities, then constraints are always open to multiple interpretations, innovations and discursive and multiple local uses by those who partake of them, whether they are qualified as powerful or powerless. Collective and organized readings and interfaces within socio-technical constraints may have regulative and/or enabling effects. If we fail to take account of this multiplicity of technological effects, we may obscure some of the mediated/active paths from which we can insurrect or disrupt them, thereby reproducing aspects of what we seek to change.

The body

Such debates connect with different understandings of the body and its writing technologies. They placed our tensions and intersections, so that on the one hand, they parallelled those around a feminist politics of identity which worried about losing the notion of the body and its political relevance; on the other, they linked with postmodernist analyses which depict the body as socio-technically constituted by many contradictory cultural images, interfaces and codes. According to the former, the malleability and mutability of the (technophilic) body may lead to the body being forgotten without recognition of its limited spaces; the latter suggests that body categories are determined by material and social conditions.

By ignoring the body, postmodernists seemed to some of us to subscribe to a conservative liberal pluralism and/or constructivist relativism. However, we also consider that where an analysis of concrete dynamics highlights the socio-technological inscriptions of the body, this does not necessarily imply a forgetting of embodied politics or celebrating its disappearance in the midst of a postmodernist flow. By contrast, we might attend to the processes of displacement and replacement, reformulation, re-presentation and/or translation of body matters and the discursive-material technologies which make it possible.

While there are already some attempts to deploy a discursive analysis of technologies within psychological research (Figueroa-Sarriera, 1993; Burman *et al.*, 1995; Gordo-López, 1995a; Parker, 1996), little attention has been paid to the ways new forms of subjectivity, communication and regulation/ resistance are associated with the design, implementation and technological policies in (medical and psychological) institutional settings. Discursive-analytical work has repeatedly repressed and displaced the significance of the technological aspects of regulatory forms. The panopticon discussed by Foucault was not a metaphor for surveillance; it was a material technology which was used to structure the architectural layout of disciplinary institutions and thus became a means of (self) regulation of the (deviant and then normalizing) self. The material and discursive dimension which inexorably accompanies the panopticon as a material and metaphorical device serves to exemplify the way the 'Eye of Power' is habitually undetachable from its visualizing technologies. Social constructionism and discursive-analytical work has often differed from, or repressed, the fact that technologies (whether architectural, informatic, experimental or surgical techniques) are also discursive artefacts in their (psychological) context of design and use. Giving voice to discursive understandings of technological actors and their interfaces with other social agencies may prompt other readings of the discursive dynamics which fix the designs and uses of technical advances (e.g. surgical advances for male-to-female sex reassignment, or other reproductive technological practices which maintain the traditional notion of the heterosexual family) and limit other possible ones (e.g. phalloplasty, third-sex positions in gender-reassignment programmes, transhomosexuality, lesbian mothers' 'parental rights').

We argue that interventionist work in the social sciences should take the content of technology seriously and in detail as a resource to critically examine the technical attributes and forms of relations between humans and technical artefacts (whether of transsexualism or the dissemination of discourses of depression in the social imaginary). These approaches give due attention to the double meaning of technologies as: 1) technologies of power (discourse); and 2) the material technologies (discursive hardware). This double understanding of technologies shifts the analysis from examination of the workings of the 'psy complex' (Ingleby, 1985; Rose, 1985) to 'psy-techno-complexes'.

From the study of specific settings in this book we have put forward analytical notions such as boundary objects which do not separate technologies from the heterogeneous networks that surround them, including the human body.

Coalitions as frictional platforms for resistance (and pleasure)

In this book tensions and disagreements have not been subordinated to a clear, coherent co-authored agenda. The suppression of tensions in this book and explicitly in these postscripts would not have done justice to the complexities and multiple experiences of its authors and their different theoretical resources. Moreover, it would have rendered our interventional alliances more vulnerable to recuperation by other more flexible coalitions, such as those which inform dominant psychological apparatuses, relations, paradoxes and technologies. By positioning our analyses between apparently diammetrically different trends and agendas we may perhaps avoid locating our studies (and those we speak on behalf of) at the level of commodities, depriving them of their relational potentials to facilitate new coalitions and heterogeneous alliances, such as the one this book has produced. The internal variability in our texts and of our contextually and politically interpellated subjectivities injects many, often overlapping and frictional, platforms of resistance into the complexity of the psychological nets.

Moving now from commenting on the theoretical importance of technologies to our process of creating this book as a technical artefact; this book was produced over a two-year period and after much trawling through the gatekeeping process of publishers' reviews. Our meetings were characterized by debates, conflicts and tensions that were sometimes inspiringly insightful and sometimes difficult – including the initial discussion on which these postscripts are based. In addition to all the other differences – between us and between us and you – we should point out that as a group we were composed of students and professionals and that the book correspondingly represents different opportunities and arenas of engagement for each of us. For all of us writing here, at some level it figures within the entry into, or maintenance of, credibility in academic life and the accumulation of cultural capital this requires (although writing books, or chapters in books, counts little in psychology because, in its emulation of science, only journal articles are valued). But beyond this, for some it has also represented a welcome space to reflect on and engage with professional practices in a different way; and to develop new tools and alternative power/knowledges from a privileged and credible arena to initiate change (for example within in-service training, see e.g. Billington, 1995; Marks *et al.*, 1995).

However, the non-homogeneity of this book is more, and more significant than, the mere accumulation of differences arising from particular institutional and professional positions. Our commonalities arose from our commitment to change and our critique of traditional psychological practices. But the discontinuities between the chapters of this book also illuminate those absences wrought by traditional psychology. Psychology has storied us and our tales of regulation and resistance out of being and, like our topics, has rendered these accounts either invisible or pathological. Our practice in this book, then, is an instance of our resistance, our refusal to collude in maintaining the practice of psychology as the reproduction of oppression (including our own). It is also an instance of our regulation or collusion, in so far as putting our politics into more academic form involves an investment in cultural capital that could divert energy or attention from more direct intervention. We can only recognize the temptations to become dogmatic and censorious of others that have also entered our own discussions.

Nevertheless, we see ourselves as doing something that is more than merely academic, in three ways. First, we are developing intellectual tools that can be mobilized for practitioners and users of services, both individually and in training. Second, our work in this book is informed by our activities outside it – as a group within the Discourse Unit and Psychology Politics Resistance and through our individual political involvements, affiliations and constituencies. Third, we want to point out how the form of this book, as a co-authored text, grinds against the grain of traditional academic practice. It disturbs the rational, unitary, omnipotent author and encourages diverse ways of reading and writing. We want to portray our ideas and academic work as jointly constructed and shared, not in the sense of uniform distribution, but of multiple perspectives that are brought together into some – albeit provisional and temporary – alliance. Hence in this book the author as a single, disembodied voice is shown to be a fiction, but the notion of authorship, in the sense of creating a story together, is very much alive; the author may be dead, but we can create different, active and embodied forms of speech.

It would be misleading, however, to allow the process of producing this book to sound as if it was all dismal struggle and argument. In terms of Barthes' notion of the pleasure of the text (Barthes, 1975), we have enjoyed the thrill and tension of this academic critique; we have all found it an exciting as well as an exercising project. We have enjoyed developing and sharing our transgressive positions on the fringes of psychology. Moreover, we do not see ourselves as involved in a solely negative or reactive project. We are building our own institutions, even as this book is a record of one, albeit short-lived and now (by the time you read it) dismantled, but with, we hope, enduring consequences.

The authors

GILL AITKEN is a trainee Clinical Psychologist at Manchester University. She was formerly Lecturer in Social Psychology at Humberside University. Her PhD (1989) was on the topic of interpersonal communication between stutterers and non-stutterers.

PAM ALLDRED was a Research Assistant on a 'Children and Families' project at the Department of Sociology, University of East London, from which she is co-author of various conference papers and reports. She is currently lecturing part-time at South Bank University and the University of East London while completing her doctoral research. In addition to other conference papers, she also co-authored *Challenging Women*, 1996, Open University Press.

ROBIN ALLWOOD is a research student at the Discourse Unit, Department of Psychology and Speech Pathology, the Manchester Metropolitan University.

TOM BILLINGTON works as an Educational Psychologist on Merseyside, having previously taught in schools and colleges for many years. He has published journal articles on the contradictions of using psychometric tests in assessing educational performance, and on discourse analysis.

ERICA BURMAN is Senior Lecturer in Developmental and Educational Psychology at the Discourse Unit, Department of Psychology and Speech Pathology, the Manchester Metropolitan University. Her previous publications include *Feminists and Psychological Practice*, 1990, Sage, (edited), *Discourse Analytic Research*, 1993, Routledge, (co-edited), *Deconstructing Developmental Psychology*, 1994, Routledge, *Qualitative Methods in Psychology*, 1994, Open University Press, (co-authored) and *Challenging Women*, 1996, Open University Press, (co-authored).

BRENDA GOLDBERG is a Research Assistant at the Discourse Unit, Department of Psychology and Speech Pathology, the Manchester Metropolitan

University. She also co-authored *Challenging Women*, 1996, Open University Press.

ÁNGEL JUAN GORDO LÓPEZ is Lecturer in Social Psychology at Bradford University. He is co-editor of *Psicologías, Discursos y Poder: Metodologías Cualitativas, Perspectivas Críticas (Psychologies, Discourses and Power, Qualitative Methods, Critical Perspectives)*, Visor, Madrid, 1996, co-author of *Fundamentos Evolutivas de la Educacíon Fundamentals of Development and Education*, 1993, author of *La Mujer Distribuida y sus Tecnologías: una aproximacíon discursiva (Women Organising Through Technology: a discursive approach)* to be published by Instituto de la Mujer, and a contributor to *The Cyborg Handbook*, Edited by Hables Gray, C. with Figueroa-Sarriera, H. and Mentor, S., Routledge, 1995.

COLLEEN HEENAN was a founder member of Leeds Women's Counselling and Psychotherapy Service. She is a feminist psychotherapist in private practice in Bradford, West Yorkshire and a part-time lecturer at Birkbeck College, London and Manchester Metropolitan University. She is currently completing a PhD at the Discourse Unit, Department of Psychology and Speech Pathology, the Metropolitan University of Manchester. She has published several journal articles on the topics of discourse analysis and therapy and was also a co-author of *Challenging Women*, 1996, Open University Press.

DEB MARKS is Lecturer in Disability Studies, Department of Psychotherapeutics, Sheffield University. She was a Susan Isaacs Research Fellow at the Institute of Education, University of London, 1993–4. Her journal articles and other publications are on the topics of education case conferences, school processes and discourse analysis. She also co-authored *Challenging Women*, 1996, Open University Press.

SAM WARNER is a Principal Clinical Psychologist with special responsibility for therapeutic psychological services for sexually abused children and young people at the Royal Liverpool Children's Hospital, Alder Hey, Liverpool. She trains service providers on issues of abuse and has given several conference papers on the area. She is currently completing a PhD at the Discourse Unit, Department of Psychology and Speech Pathology, the Manchester Metropolitan University, and was also co-author of *Challenging Women*, 1996, Open University Press.

References

ADVISORY CENTRE FOR EDUCATION (1992) *Findings from Advisory Centre for Education Investigations into Exclusions*, London, ACE.

AFSHAR, H. and MAYNARD, M. (1994) 'Introduction: The dynamics of 'race' and 'gender', in AFSHAR, H. and MAYNARD, M. (Eds) *The Dynamics of 'Race' and Gender*, London, Taylor & Francis.

AHMAD, W. (1992) 'Race, disadvantage and discourse: contextualising black people's health', in AHMAD, W. (Ed.) *Politics of Race and Health*, Bradford, University of Bradford Print Unit.

AHMAD, W. (1993) 'Making black people sick: "race", ideology and health research', in AHMAD, W. (Ed.) *'Race' and Health in Contemporary Britain*, Buckingham, Open University Press.

AITKEN, G. (in progress) 'The present absence of people of African–Caribbean and Asian origins within clinical, psychology services 1989–1994: A preliminary study', unpublished small-scale research project to be submitted to Department of Clinical Psychology, University of Manchester.

ALLADIN, W. J. (1992) 'Clinical psychology provision', in AHMAD, W. (Ed.) *Politics of Race and Health*, Bradford, University of Bradford Print Unit.

ALLDRED, P. (1996) 'Fit to Parent? Developmental psychology and "non-traditional" families', in BURMAN, E., ALLDRED, P. BEWLEY, E., GOLDBERG, B., HEENAN, C., MARKS, D., MARSHALL, J., TAYLOR, K., ULLAH, R. and WARNER, S. *Challenging Women: Psychology's Exclusions, Feminist Possibilities*, Buckingham, Open University Press.

ALLEN, H. (1987) *Justice Unbalanced: Gender, Psychiatry and Judicial Decisions*, Milton Keynes, Open University Press.

ALTHUSSER, L. (1971) 'Freud and Lacan', in *Lenin and Philosophy and Other Essays*, London, New Left Books.

ANDREWS, K. (1990) 'Hell on earth', paper presented at inaugural WISH conference, London.

ANON (1994) 'Why we run for cover', *WISH Newsletter*, summer, 12, London, WISH.

ANTHIAS, F. and YUVAL-DAVIS, N. with CAIN, H. (1993) *Racialised Boundaries: Race, Nation, Gender, Colour and Class and the Antiracist Struggle*, London, Routledge.

ARDITTI, R. (1982) 'Feminism and science', in WHITELEGG, E., ARNOT, M., BARTELS, E., BEECHEY, V., BIRKE, L., HIMMELWEIT, S., LEONARD, D., RUEHL, S. and SPEAKMAN, M. (Eds) *The Changing Experience of Women*, Oxford, Basil Blackwell/The Open University.

BAILEY, M. E. (1993) 'Foucauldian feminism: contesting bodies, sexuality and identity' in RAMAZANOGLU, C. (Ed.) *Up against Foucault: Explorations of some Tensions between Foucault and Feminism*, London, Routledge.

BAKER MILLER, J. (1976) *Toward a New Psychology of Women*, Harmondsworth, Pelican Books.

BAKHTIN, M. (1968) *Rabelais and his World*, Bloomington, Indiana University Press.

BALKA, E. (1993) 'Women's access to on-line discussions about feminism', *Electronic Journal of Communication*, **3**, 1, machine-readable file available through comserve@vm.its.rpi.edu.

BANISTER, P., BURMAN, E., PARKER, I., TAYLOR, M. and TINDALL, C. (1994) *Qualitative Methods in Psychology: a Research Guide*, Milton Keynes, Open University Press.

BANKS, M. and SWIFT, A. (1987) *The Joke's on Us*, London, Pandora.

BANTON, R., CLIFFORD, P., FROSH, S., LOUSANDA, J. and ROSENHALL, J. (1985) *The Politics of Mental Health*, London, Macmillan.

BARNES, M. and MAPLE, N. (1992) *Women and Mental Health: Challenging the Stereotypes*, Birmingham, Venture Press.

BARNES, M. and POTIER, M. (1993) 'Developing a research agenda for women and special hospitals: report of a workshop at Ashworth Hospital', Liverpool, unpublished.

BARRECA, R. (Ed.) (1988) *Last Laughs: Perspectives on Women and Comedy*, London, Gordon & Breach.

BARRETT, M. and MCINTOSH, M. (1982) *The Anti-Social Family*, London, New Left Books.

BARRETT, M. and TREVITT, J. (1991) *Attachment Behaviour and the Schoolchild: an Introduction to Educational Therapy*, London, Tavistock/Routledge.

BARTHES, R. (1975) *The Pleasure of the Text*, London, Jonathan Cape.

BARTHES, R. (1977) *Image-Music-Text*, London, Flamingo.

BARTKY, S. L. (1988) 'Foucault, femininity, and the modernization of patriarchal power', in DIAMOND, I. and QUINBY, L. (Eds) *Feminism and Foucault: Reflections on Resistance*, Boston, MA, Northeastern University Press.

BARTON, L. (Ed.) (1989) *Disability and Dependency*, Sussex, Falmer Press.

BARWICK, S. (1992) 'Recovering from a spell in hospital', *The Independent*, 8 August.

BEDELL, G. (1990) 'Mad, bad or just forgotten?', *The Independent on Sunday*, 4 November.

BELL, V. (1993) *Interrogating Incest: Feminism, Foucault and the Law*, London, Routledge.

BENDER, M. and RICHARDSON, A. (1990) 'The ethnic composition of clinical psychology in Britain', *The Psychologist: Bulletin of the British Psychological Society*, **6**, pp. 250–2.

BENJAMIN, H. (1966) *The Transsexual Phenomenon*, New York, Julian Press.

BENNATHAN, M. (1993) 'The care and education of troubled children', *Therapeutic Care and Education*, **1**, 1, Spring, pp. 37–49.

BERG, A.- J. and LIE, M. (1993) 'Do artifacts have gender? Feminism and the domestication of technical artifacts', *Scientific Proceedings of European Theoretical Perspectives on New Technology: Feminism, Constructivism and Utility*, West London Uxbridge, UK.

BETTELHEIM, B. and ZEHAN, K. (1982) *On Learning to Read*, London, Penguin.

BHAT, A., CARR-HILL, R. and OHRI, S. (Eds) (1988) *Britain's Black Population: A New Perspective*, Aldershot, Gower.

BHATE, S. (1987) 'Prejudice against doctors and students from ethnic minorities', *British Medical Journal*, **294**, p. 838.

BHAVNANI, K. and HARAWAY, D. (1994) 'Shifting the subject: a conversation between Kum Kum Bhavnani and Donna Haraway. 12 April 1993, Santa Cruz', *Feminism and Psychology*, **4**, 1, pp. 19–39.

BHAVNANI, K. and PHOENIX, A. (1994) 'Shifting identities, shifting racisms: an introduction', *Feminism and Psychology*, **4**, pp. 5–18.

BILLIG, M., CONDOR, S., EDWARDS, D., GANE, M., MIDDLETON, D. and RADLEY, A. (1988) *Ideological Dilemmas: a Social Psychology of Everyday Thinking*, London, Sage.

BILLINGTON, T. (1993) 'Sex differences in student estimations of female and male student–teacher interactions', *Research in Education*, **50**, November, pp. 17–26, Manchester University Press.

BILLINGTON, T. (1995) 'Discourse analysis: acknowledging interpretation in everyday practice', *Educational Psychology in Practice*, **11**, 3, pp. 36–45.

BLACK HEALTH WORKERS' AND PATIENTS' GROUP (1983) 'Psychiatry and the corporate state', *Race and Class*, **XXV**, pp. 249–64, Oxford, Blackwell.

BLAND, L. (1982) '"Guardians of the race or vampires upon the nation's health?" female sexuality and its regulation in early twentieth century Britain', in WHITELEGG, E., ARNOT, M., BARTELS, E., BEECHEY, V., BIRKE, L., HIMMELWEIT, S., LEONARD, D., RUEHL, S. and SPEAKMAN, M. (Eds) *The Changing Experience of Women*, Oxford: Basil Blackwell/The Open University.

BONDI, L. (1993) 'Locating identity politics', in KEITT, M. and PILE, J. (Eds) *Place and the Politics of Identity*, London, Routledge.

BOOTH, H. (1988) 'Identifying ethnic origin: the past, present and future of official data production', in BHAT, A., CARR-HILL, R. and OHRI, S. (Eds) (1988) *Britain's Black Population: A New Perspective*, Aldershot, Gower.

BORDO, S. (1988) 'Anorexia nervosa: psychopathology as the crystallization of culture', in DIAMOND, I. and QUINBY, L. (Eds) *Feminism and Foucault: Reflections on Resistance*, Boston MA, Northeastern University Press.

BORDO, S. (1992) 'Anorexia nervosa: psychopathology as the crystallization of culture', in CROWLEY, H. and HIMMELWEIT, S. (Eds) *Knowing Women: Feminism and Knowledge*, Milton Keynes, Open University Press.

BOURDIEU, P. and WACQUANT, L. (1992) *An Invitation to Reflexive Sociology*, Chicago IL, University of Chicago Press.

BOWERS, J. and MIDDLETON, D. (1992) 'Distributed organizational cognition: an innovative idea?', in TURNER, W. (Ed.) *The Management of Intellectual Resources*, Paris, Economica.

BOWLBY, J. (1973) *Attachment and Loss, Vol. 2, 'Separation: Anxiety and Anger'*, London, Hogarth Press.

BOYLE, M. (1992) *Deconstructing Schizophrenia*, London, Routledge.

BRAH, A. (1991) 'Questions of difference and international feminism', in AARON, J. and WAALBY, S. (Eds) *Out of the Margins: Women's Studies in the Nineties*, London, The Falmer Press.

BRAH, A. (1992) 'Difference, diversity and differentiation', in DONALD, J. and RATTANSI, A. (Eds) *'Race', Culture and Difference*, Buckingham, Open University Press/Sage.

BRODRIBB, S. (1992) *Nothing Mat(t)ers: a Feminist Critique of Postmodernism*, Melbourne, Spinifex.

BROE, M. L. (1987) *Silence and Power: Djuna Barnes, A Revaluation*, Carbondale IL, University of Southern Illinois Press.

BROOKNER, A. (1994) 'The death of innocence', *The Observer*, 6 March.

BROVERMAN, I., BROVERMAN, D., CLARKSON, F., ROSENKRANTZ, P. and VOGEL, S. (1970) 'Sex-role stereotypes and clinical judgements of mental health', *Journal of Consulting and Clinical Psychology*, **34**, pp. 1–7.

BROWNE, D. (1990) *Black People, Mental Health and the Courts*, London, National Association for the Care and Resettlement of Offenders (NACRO).

BURMAN, E. (1991a) 'What discourse is not', *Philosophical Psychology*, **5**, 3, pp. 325–42.

BURMAN, E. (1991b) 'Power, gender and developmental psychology', *Feminism and Psychology*, **1**, 1, pp. 141–53.

BURMAN, E. (1992) 'Identification and power in feminist therapy – a reflexive history of a discourse analysis', *Women's Studies International Forum*, **15**, 4, pp. 487–98.

BURMAN, E. (1994a) *Deconstructing Developmental Psychology*, London, Routledge.

BURMAN, E. (1994b) 'Experience, identities and alliances: Jewish feminism and feminist psychology', in BHAVNANI, K. and PHOENIX, A. (Eds) *Shifting Identities, Shifting Racism: a Feminism and Psychology Reader*, **4**, 1, pp. 155–78.

BURMAN, E. (1994c) 'Innocents abroad: Western fantasies of childhood and the iconography of emergencies', *Disasters: The Journal of Disaster Studies and Management*, **18**, 3, pp. 238–54.

BURMAN, E. (1995) 'Identification, subjectivity and change in feminist therapy', in SIEGFRIED, J. (Ed.) *Therapeutic and Everyday Discourse as Behavior Change*, New York, Ablex.

BURMAN, E. (1996) '"The crisis in modern social psychology and how to find it": Discourses of discourse in psychological research methods', *South African Journal of Psychology*, **26**, 3, pp. 1–8.

BURMAN, E., GORDO LÓPEZ, A. J., MACAULEY, W. R. and PARKER, I. (1995) (Eds) *Cyberpsychology: Conference, Interventions and Reflections*, Manchester, Discourse Unit, Manchester Metropolitan University.

BURMAN, E. and PARKER, I. (1993) (Eds) *Discursive Analytic Research: Repertories and Readings of Texts in Action*, London, Routledge.

BUTLER, J. (1990a) 'Gender trouble, feminist theory, and psychoanalytic discourse', in NICHOLSON, L. J. (Ed.) *Feminism/Postmodernism*, New York, Routledge.

BUTLER, J. (1990b) *Gender Trouble: Feminism and the Subversion of Identity*, London, Routledge.

BUTLER, J. (1992) 'Contingent foundations: feminism and the question of postmodernism', in BUTLER, J. and SCOTT, J. (Eds) *Feminists Theorise the Political*, London, Routledge.

BUTLER, J. (1993a) *Bodies That Matter: On the Discursive Limits of 'Sex'*, London, Routledge.

BUTLER, J. (1993b) 'Gender as performance: an interview with Judith Butler', *Radical Philosophy*, **68**, pp. 32–9.

CALLON, M. (1991) 'Techno-economic networks and irreversibility', in LAW, J. (Ed.) *A Sociology of Monsters: Essays on Power, Technology and Domination*, London, Routledge.

CAPLAN, P. and GANS, M. (1991) 'Is there empirical justification for the category of "self-defeating personality disorder"?', *Feminism and Psychology*, **1**, pp. 263–78.

CARR-HILL, R. and DREW, D. (1988) 'Blacks, police and crime', in BHAT, A., CARR-HILL, R. and OHRI, S. (Eds) (1988) *Britain's Black Population: A New Perspective*, Aldershot, Gower.

CASEMENT, P. (1985) *On Learning from the Patient*, London, Tavistock/Routledge.

CASEMENT, P. (1990) *Further Learning from the Patient – The Analytic Space and Process*, London, Tavistock/Routledge.

CHAN, M. (1995) 'The NHS response to minority ethnic health: improving services for Asian people with learning disabilities', presentation at a one-day event for Asian staff, University of Manchester, April.

(CHARLES) HELEN (1992) 'Whiteness: The relevance of politically colouring the "non"', in HINDS, H., PHOENIX, A. and STACEY, J. (Eds) *Working Out, New Directions for Women's Studies*, London, The Falmer Press.

CHATTERJEE, D. (1995) 'Harnessing Shakti: the work of the Bengali Women's Support Group', in GRIFFIN, G. (Ed.) *Feminist Activism in the 1990s*, London, Taylor & Francis.

CHAUDHURI, N. and STROBEL, M. (Eds) (1992) *Western Women and Imperialism – Complicity and Resistance*, Bloomington, IN, Indiana University Press.

CHEAL, D. (1991) *Family and the State of Theory*, Hemel Hempstead, Harvester Wheatsheaf.

CHESLER, P. (1972) *Women and Madness*, New York, Doubleday.

CHODOROW, N. (1978) *The Reproduction of Mothering: Psychoanalysis and the Sociology of Gender*, Berkeley, CA, University of California Press.

CHODOROW, N. (1989) *Feminism and Psychoanalytic Theory*, New Haven, CT, Yale University Press.

CHODOROW, N. (1994) *Femininities, Masculinities, Sexualities – Freud and Beyond*, London, Free Association Press.

COCKBURN, C. and FÜRST-DILI, R. (Eds) (1994) *Bringing Technology Home: Gender and Technology in a Changing Europe*, Milton Keynes, Open University Press.

COHEN, P. (1988) 'The perversions of inheritance', in COHEN, P. and BAINS, H. (Eds) *Multi-Racist Britain*, Basingstoke, Macmillan Education.

COLLIER, S. and DIBBLIN, J. (1990) 'Justice weighted against women', *The Observer*, 28 October.

COLLINS, P. (1990) *Black Feminist Thought: Knowledge, Consciousness and the Politics of Empowerment*, London, HarperCollins Academic.

COOTER, R. (Ed.) (1992) *In the Name of the Child*, London, Routledge.

COWARD, R. (1989) *The Whole Truth: The Myth of Alternative Health*, London, Faber & Faber.

CREED, B. (Winter, 1987) 'Horror and the monstrous-feminine: an imaginary abjection', *Screen*, **28**, 1, pp. 44–70.

CULLINGFORD, C. (1991) *The Inner World of the School: Children's Ideas about School*, London, Cassell Education.

CURT, B. (1994) *Textuality and Tectonics*, Milton Keynes, Open University Press.

DALY, M. (1979) *Gyn/ecology: the metaethics of radical feminism*, London, Women's Press.

DAVIE, R., PHILLIPS, D. and CALLELY, E. (1984) *Evaluation of INSET Course on Behaviour Problems*, Report to Welsh Office, Cardiff, Department of Education, University College.

DAVIES, L. (1984) *Pupil Power: Gender and Deviance*, Hove, Falmer Press.

DAVIES, P. (1990) 'A woman in all but legal nicety', *The Independent*, 20 April, p. 17.

DAVIS, N. Z. (1965) *Society and Culture in Early Modern France*, Stanford, CA, Stanford University Press.

DE LAURETIS, T. (1989) *Technologies of Gender: Essays on Theory, Film and Fiction*, Basingstoke, Macmillan.

DEPARTMENT FOR EDUCATION AND SCIENCE (DFE) (1994) *Code of Practice: on the identification and assessment of special educational needs*, London, Central Office of Information.

DEPARTMENT OF EDUCATION AND SCIENCE (DES) (1978) *Special Educational Needs*, (Warnock Report), Cmnd 7212, London, HMSO.

DEPARTMENT OF HEALTH (1993a) *The Health of the Nation: Mental Illness*, London, DOH.

DEPARTMENT OF HEALTH (1993b) *Ethnicity and Health: A Guide for the NHS*, London, DOH.

DERRIDA, J. (1973) *Speech and Phenomena, and Other Essays on Husserl's Theory of Signs*, Evanston, IL, Northwestern University Press.

DERRIDA, J. (1976) *Of Grammatology*, Baltimore MD, Johns Hopkins University Press.

DIAMOND, I. and QUINBY, L. (Eds) (1988) *Feminism and Foucault: Reflections on Resistance*, Boston, MA, Northeastern University Press.

DIANE (1994) 'Why did I lose my son?', *WISH (Women in Special Hospitals) Newsletter*, summer, 7, London, WISH.

DINNERSTEIN, D. (1976) *The Rocking of the Cradle and the Ruling of the World*, London, Souvenir Press.

DOLLIMORE, J. (1991) *Sexual Dissidence: Augustine to Wilde, Freud to Foucault*, Oxford, Clarendon Press.

DONALD, J. and RATTANSI, A. (Eds) (1992) *'Race', Culture and Difference*, London, Sage.

DONOVAN, J. (1991) *Feminist Theory: The Intellectual Traditions of American Feminism*, New York, Continuum.

DONZELOT, J. (1980) *The Policing of Families: Welfare Versus the State*, London, Hutchinson.

DUDEN, B. (1992) 'Populations', in SACHS, W. (Ed.) *The Development Dictionary: a Guide to Knowledge as Power*, London, Zed Press.

DUGGER, K. (1991) 'Social location and gender-role attitudes: a comparison of black and white women', in LORBER, J. and FARRELL, S. (Eds) *The Social Construction of Gender*, Beverly Hills, CA, Sage.

DUTTON-DOUGLAS, M. A. and WALKER, L. E. (Eds) (1988) *Feminist Psychotherapies: Integration of Therapeutic and Feminist Systems*. Norwood, NJ, Ablex.

DYER, G. (1994) 'Journey to the heart of darkness', *The Guardian*, 12 March.

EAGLETON, T. (1981) *Walter Benjamin, or, Towards a Revolutionary Criticism*, London, Verso.

EAGLETON, T. (1989) 'Bakhtin, Schopenhauer, Kundera', in HIRSCHKOP, K. and SHEPHERD, D. (Eds) *Bakhtin and Cultural Theory*, Manchester, Manchester University Press.

EDWARDS, D. and MIDDLETON, D. (1988) 'Conversational remembering and family relationships: how children learn to remember', *Journal of Social and Personal Relationships*, **5**, pp. 1–25.

EHRENREICH, B. and ENGLISH, D. (1979) *For Her Own Good: 150 Years of the Experts' Advice to Women*, London, Pluto Press.

EICHENBAUM, L. and ORBACH, S. (1982) *Outside In, Inside Out: Women's*

Psychology – A Feminist Psychoanalytic Approach, Harmondsworth, Pelican Books.

EICHENBAUM, L. and ORBACH, S. (1983) *What Do Women Want?* London, Fontana.

EICHENBAUM, L. and ORBACH, S. (1987) 'Separation and intimacy', in ERNST, S. and MAGUIRE, L. (Eds) *Living with the Sphinx: Papers from the Women's Therapy Centre*, London, Women's Press.

ELAM, D. (1994) *Feminism and Deconstruction: Ms en Abyme*, London, Routledge.

ELLIS, M. L. (1994) 'Lesbian, gay men and psychoanalytic training', *Free Associations*, **4**, 32, pp. 501–17.

ELSHTAIN, J. B. (1982) 'Feminist discourse and its discontents: language, power, and meaning', *Signs: Journal of Women in Culture and Society*, **7**, 3, pp. 603–21.

ERNST, S. (1987) 'Can a daughter be a woman?' in ERNST, S. and MAGUIRE, L. (Eds) *Living with the Sphinx: Papers from the Women's Therapy Centre*, London, Women's Press.

ESSED, P. (1991) *Understanding Everyday Racism: An Interdisciplinary Theory*, London, Sage.

EVANS, D. T. (1993) *The Sexual Citizenship: The Material Construction of Sexualities*, London and New York, Routledge.

FARMER, B. and McGUFFIN, P. (1989) 'The classification of the depressions: contemporary confusion revisited', *British Journal of Psychiatry*, **155**, pp. 437–43.

FEATHERSTONE, M. (1991) 'The body in consumer culture', in FEATHERSTONE, M., HEPWORTH, M. and TURNER, B. S. (Eds) *The Body: Social Process and Cultural Theory*, London, Sage.

FERNANDO, S. (1991) *Race, Culture and Mental Health*, Basingstoke, Macmillan.

FERNANDO, S. (1993a) 'Psychiatry and racism', *Changes*, **11**, pp. 46–58.

FERNANDO, S. (1993b) 'Racial bias and schizophrenia', *Transcultural Psychiatry Society Bulletin*, **2**, pp. 9–13.

FIGUEROA-SARRIERA, H. (1993) 'Some body fantasies in cyberspace text: a view from its exclusions', paper presented at the International Conference for Theoretical Psychology, Saclas, France, April.

FIRESTONE, S. (1970) *The Dialectic of Sex: The Case for Feminist Revolution*, New York, William Morrow.

FLAX, J. (1990) *Thinking Fragments: Psychoanalysis, Feminism, and Postmodernism in the Contemporary West*, Berkeley, CA, University of California Press.

FLAX, J. (1993) *Disputed Subjects: Essays on Psychoanalysis, Politics and Philosophy*, New York, Routledge.

FORD, J., MONGON, D. and WHELAN, M. (1982) *Special Education and Social Control*, London, Routledge & Kegan Paul.

References

FLYNN, J. R. (1989) 'Rushton, evolution and race: An essay on intelligence and virtue', *The Psychologist*, **2**, 9, pp. 363–6.

FOUCAULT, M. (1961) *Madness and Civilisation: A History of Insanity in the Age of Reason*, London, Routledge.

FOUCAULT, M. (1973) *The Birth of the Clinic*, London, Tavistock.

FOUCAULT, M. (1977a) *Discipline and Punish: The Birth of the Prison*, Harmondsworth, Penguin Books.

FOUCAULT, M. (1977b) *Language, Counter-Memory, Practice: Selected Essays and Interviews*, Oxford, Blackwell.

FOUCAULT, M. (1979a) 'On governmentality', *Ideology and Consciousness*, **6**, pp. 5–22.

FOUCAULT, M. (1979b) *The History of Sexuality. Vol. I: An Introduction*, London, Allen Lane.

FOUCAULT, M. (1980a) *Power/Knowledge: Selected Interviews and Other Writings 1972–1977*, Hassocks, Sussex, Harvester Press.

FOUCAULT, M. (1980b) 'Truth and power', in FOUCAULT, M. *Power/Knowledge*, Brighton, Harvester Press.

FOUCAULT, M. (1981) 'The order of discourse', in YOUNG, R. (Ed.) *Untying the Text*, London, Routledge.

FOUCAULT, M. (1982) 'The subject and power', in DREYFUS, H. and RABINOW, P. *Beyond Structuralism and Hermeneutics*, Chicago IL, Chicago University Press.

FOUCAULT, M. (1985) *Herculine Barbine Llamada Alexina B*, SERRANO, A. (Ed.), Introduction by M. FOUCAULT, 'El Sexo Verdadero', pp. 11–20, Madrid, Revolución.

FOUCAULT, M. (1992) *Microfisica del Poder*, VARELA, J. and ÁLVAREZ-URÍA, F. (Eds and trans.), 3rd Edn, Madrid, La Piqueta.

FRASER, N. (1989) *Unruly Practices: Power, Discourse and Gender in Contemporary Social Theory*, Cambridge, Polity Press.

FREUD, S. (1986) in FREUD, A. (Ed.) *The Essentials of Psychoanalysis*, Harmondsworth, Pelican Books.

FRIEDMAN, S. and HARRISON, G. (1984) 'Sexual histories, attitudes and behaviour of schizophrenic and "normal" women', *Archives of Sexual Behaviour*, **13**, pp. 555–67.

FROMM, E. (1979) *To Have or To Be?*, London, Sphere.

FROSH, S. (1987) *The Politics of Psychoanalysis*, London, Macmillan.

FROSH, S. (1989) *Psychoanalysis and Psychology: Minding the Gap*, London, Macmillan Education.

GARBER, M. (1992) *Vested Interest: Cross-dressing and Cultural Anxiety*, New York, Routledge.

GAVEY, N. (1989) 'Feminist poststructuralism and discourse analysis – contributions to feminist psychology', *Psychology of Women Quarterly*, **13**, pp. 459–75.

GERGEN, K. (1989) 'Warranting voice and the elaboration of self', in SHOTTER, J. and GERGEN, K. (Eds) *Texts of Identity*, London, Sage.

GERGEN, K., GLOGER-TIPPELT, G. and BERKOWITZ, P. (1990) 'The cultural construction of the developing child', in SEMIN, G. and GERGEN, K. (Eds) *Everyday Understanding: Social and Scientific Implications*, London, Sage.

GERSCH, I. S. and NOLAN, A. (1994) 'Exclusions: what the children think', *Educational Psychology in Practice*, **10**, 1, April.

GILBERT, P. (1992) *Depression: The Evolution of Powerlessness*, Hove, Lawrence Erlbaum Associates.

GILMAN, S. (1992) 'Black bodies, white bodies: towards an iconography of female sexuality in late nineteenth-century art, medicine and literature', in DONALD, J. and RATTANSI, A. (Eds) *'Race', Culture and Difference*, Buckingham, Open University Press/Sage.

GOOD, B. J. (1994) *Medicine, Rationality and Experience, An Anthropological Perspective*, Cambridge, Cambridge University Press.

GORDO LÓPEZ, A. J. (1994) 'Gender identity clinic rhetorics: developmental knowledge on gender identities and other boundary objects', presentation at the Bristish Psychological Society, Developmental Psychological Section Conference, Portsmouth University, Portsmouth, UK, September.

GORDO LÓPEZ, A. J. (1995a) 'Gendered psycho-techno-complexes: the dynamics of boundary objects', unpublished PhD thesis, University of Manchester.

GORDO LÓPEZ, A. J. (1995b) 'Introduction' to the Symposium 'Cyberpsychology: Discursive Approaches to the PsyÄTechnoÄComplex', presentation at The International Conference Understanding the Social World: Towards an Integrative Approach, The University of Huddersfield, UK, June.

GORDO LÓPEZ, A. J. and GEORGACA, E. (1993) 'Reporting-acts and discursive artifacts: a performative analysis of linguistic practices on gender and sexuality', presentation at the International Society for Theoretical Psychology Conference, Saclas, France, April.

GORDO LÓPEZ, A. J. and LINAZA, J. L. (1995) 'Introduction', in GORDO LÓPEZ, A. J. and LINAZA, J. L. (Eds) *Psicologías, Discursos y Poder (PDP)*, Madrid, Visor.

GORDON, P. (1993) 'Keeping therapy white?: psychotherapy trainings and equal opportunities', *British Journal of Psychotherapy*, **10**, pp. 44–9.

GREEN, R. (1987) *The 'Sissy Boy Syndrome' and the Development of Homosexuality*, New Haven, CT, Yale University Press.

GRIFFIN, G. (1995) 'The struggle continues – an interview with Hannana Siddiqui of Southall Black Sisters', in GRIFFIN, G. (Ed.) *Feminist Activism in the 1990s*, London, Taylor & Francis,

GROSZ, E. (1989) *Sexual Subversions: Three French Feminists*, Sydney, Allen & Unwin.

HARAWAY, D. (1991) *Simians, Cyborgs, and Women: The Reinvention of Nature*, London, Free Association Press.

References

HARDYMENT, C. (1983) *Dream Babies: Childcare from Locke to Spock*, London, Jonathan Cape.

HARE-MUSTIN, R. T. (1980) 'Psychotherapy and women – priorities for research', in BRODSKY, A. M. and HARE-MUSTIN, R. T. (Eds) *Women and Psychotherapy – An Assessment of Research and Practice*, New York, Guilford Press.

HARE-MUSTIN, R. T. and MARACEK, J. (1990) 'Gender and the meaning of difference: postmodernism and psychology', in HARE-MUSTIN, R. T. and MARACEK, J. (Eds) *Making a Difference*, New Haven, CT, Yale University Press.

HARRÉ, R. and SECORD, P. (1972) *The Explanation of Social Behaviour*, Oxford, Blackwell.

HEALTH JOURNAL (1989) 'Working for patients: new diagnosis–new presciption', *The Health Journal*, 2 February.

HEAP, E. (1975) 'The supervisor as reflector', *Social Work Today*, **5**, 22, pp. 677–9.

HEATH, S. (1986) 'Joan Riviere and the masquerade', in BURGIN, V., DONALD, J. and KAPLAN, C. (Eds) *Formations of Fantasy*, London, Methuen.

HEENAN, M. C. (1995a) 'Feminist psychotherapy – a contradiction in terms?', *Feminism and Psychology*, **5**, 1, pp. 112–17.

HEENAN, M. C. (1995b) 'Women, food and fat: too many cooks in the kitchen?', in BURMAN, E., ALLDRED, P., BEWLEY, C., GOLDBERG, B., HEENAN, M. C., MARKS, D., MARSHALL, J., TAYLOR, K., ULLAH, R. and WARNER, S. *Challenging Women: Psychology's Exclusions, Feminist Possibilities*, Buckingham, Open University Press.

HENRIQUES, J., HOLLWAY, W., URWIN, C., VENN, C. and WALKERDINE, V. (1984) *Changing the Subject: Psychology, Social Regulation and Subjectivity*, London, Methuen.

HMSO (1992a) *Report of the committee of inquiry into complaints about Ashworth Hospital: volume one*, London, HMSO.

HMSO (1992b) *Report of the committee of inquiry into complaints about Ashworth Hospital: volume two – the case studies*, London, HMSO.

HOLLWAY, W. (1989) *Subjectivity and Method in Psychology: Gender, Meaning and Science*, London, Sage.

HOWARTH, A. (1994) 'Sex in Japan', *Marie Claire*, **10**, June, pp. 10–20.

HOYLES, M. and EVANS, P. (1989) *The Politics of Childhood*, London, Journeyman Press.

HUNT, J. (1983) 'Psychoanalytic aspects of fieldwork', *Sage University Paper Series on Qualitative Research Methods*, **1**, Beverly Hills, CA, Sage.

HUNT, P.(1994) *Working Across Cultures: Catering for Whose Needs: Is Change Needed?* London, St George's Mental Health Library Conference Series.

IBÁÑEZ, T. (1995) 'Construccionismo y Psicología', in GORDO LÓPEZ, A. J. and LINAZA, J. L. (Eds) *Psicologías, Discursos y Poder (PDP)*, Madrid, Visor.

INGLEBY, D. (1985) 'Professionals as socializers: the "psy complex"', *Research in Law, Deviance and Social Control*, **7**, pp. 16–24, 79–109.

IRIGARAY, L. (1985) *This Sex That is Not One*, New York, Cornell University Press.

JACKSON, S. (1992) 'The amazing deconstructing woman', *Trouble and Strife*, **25**, Winter.

JAMES, A. and PROUT, A. (Eds) (1990) *Constructing and Reconstructing Childhood*, London, Falmer Press.

KANDO, T. (1973) *Sex Change: The Achievement of Gender Identity among Feminized Transsexuals*, Springfield, IL, Charles C. Thomas.

KAPLAN, E. A. (1992) *Motherhood and Representation: The Mother in Popular Culture and Melodrama*, London, Routledge.

KEGAN GARDINER, J. (1992) 'Psychoanalysis and feminism: an American humanist's view', *Signs: Journal of Women in Culture and Society*, **17**, 2, pp. 437–54.

KELLY, A. (1988) 'Gender differences in teacher–pupil interaction: a meta-analytic review', *Research in Education*, **39**, pp. 1–23, Manchester University Press.

KENNEDY, H. (1993) *Eve was Framed: Women and British Justice*, London, Vintage Books.

KITZINGER, C. and PERKINS, R. (1993) *Changing Our Minds – Lesbian Feminism and Psychology*, London, Only Women Press.

KLEIN, M. (1976) 'Feminist concepts of therapy outcome', *Psychotherapy: Theory, Research and Practice*, **13**, 1, pp. 89–95.

KLEIN, M. (1988) *Envy and Gratitude and Other Works 1946–1963*, London, Virago.

KLEIN, M.(1989) *The Psychoanalysis of Children*, London, Virago.

KOHLBERG, L. (1969) 'The Child as Moral Philosopher', in SANTS, J. (Ed.) *Developmental Psychology*, Harmondsworth, Penguin.

KRISTEVA, J. (1982) *Powers of Horror*, New York, Columbia University Press.

KVALE, S. (Ed.) (1992) *Psychology and Postmodernism*, London, Sage.

LAIDLAW, T. A., MALMO, C. and associates (1990) *Healing Voices: Feminist Approaches to Therapy with Women*, San Francisco, CA, Jossey-Bass Publishers.

LANGS, R. J. (1980) 'Supervision and the bipersonal field', in HESS, A. K. (Ed.) *Psychotherapy Supervision: Theory, Research and Practice*, New York, J. Wiley.

LATOUR, B. (1986) 'The power of association', in LAW, J. (Ed.) *Power, Action and Belief: A New Sociology of Knowledge? Sociological Review Monograph*, 32, London, Routledge & Kegan Paul.

LATOUR, B. (1988) *The Pasteurization of France Followed by Reductions*, SHERIDAN, A. and LAW, J. (trans.) Cambridge, MA, Harvard University Press.

LAW, J. (1992) 'Notes on the theory of the actor-network: ordering, strategy and heterogeneity', *System Practices*, **5**, pp. 379–93.

References

LAWRENCE, M. (Ed.) (1987) *Fed Up and Hungry: Women, Oppression and Food*, London, Women's Press.

LEONARD, P. (1984) *Personality and Ideology: Towards a Materialist Understanding of the Individual*, London, Macmillan.

LEWIN, E. (1994) 'Negotiating lesbian motherhood: the dialectics of resistance and accommodation', in NAKANO GLENN, E., CHANG, G. and RENNIE FORCEY, L. (Eds) *Mothering: Ideology, Experience, Agency*, London, Routledge.

LIDDLE, J. and RAI, S. M. (1993) 'Between feminism and orientalism', in KENNEDY, M., LUBELSKA, C. and WALSH, V. (Eds) *Making Connections*, London, Taylor & Francis.

LITTLEWOOD, R. (1991) 'Against pathology: the new psychiatry and its critics', *British Journal of Psychiatry*, **159**, pp. 696–702.

LITTLEWOOD, R. (1993) 'Ideology, camouflage or contingency? racism in British psychiatry', *Transcultural Psychiatric Research Review*, **30**, pp. 243–90.

LITTLEWOOD, R. and LIPSEDGE, M. (1988) 'Psychiatric illness among British Afro–Caribbeans', *British Medical Journal*, **296**, pp. 950–1.

LITTLEWOOD, R. and LIPSEDGE, M. (1989) *Aliens and Alienists: Ethnic Minorities and Psychiatry (2E)*, London, Unwin Hyman.

LIVINGSTON SMITH, D. (1991) *Hidden Conversations: An Introduction to Communicative Psychoanalysis*, London, Routledge.

LLOYD, A. (1991) 'Women: altered states', *The Guardian*, 25 January.

LLOYD, A. (1995). *Doubly Deviant, Doubly Damned: Society's Treatment of Violent Women*, Harmondsworth, Penguin Books.

LONSDALE, S. (1993) 'When sex-change is a mistake', *The Independent*, 24 October, p. 25.

LOTHSTEIN, L. M. (1983) *Female-to-Male Transsexualism: Historical, Clinical and Theoretical Issues*, Boston, MA, Routledge.

MACAULEY, W. R. and GORDO-LÓPEZ, A. J. (1995) 'From cognitive psychologies to mythologies: advancing cyborg textualities for a narrative of resistance', in GRAY, C. H., FIGUEROA-SARRIERA, H. J. and MENTOR, S. (Eds) *The Cyborg Handbook*, London and New York, Routledge.

MACCARTHY, B. (1988) 'Clinical work with ethnic minorities', in WATTS, F. (Ed.) *New Developments in Clinical Psychology*, **2**, BPS/John Wiley.

MCINTYRE, K. (1994) 'Time for action now: the African–Caribbean perspective', in National Health Service Task Force *Time for Action Now – Regional Race Programme: Greater Manchester Seminar*, London, Department of Health.

MCLEOD, E. (1994) *Women's Experiences of Feminist Therapy and Counselling*, Buckingham, Open University Press.

MCNAY, L. (1992) *Feminism and Foucault*, Oxford, Polity Press.

MAHONEY, M. A. and YNGVESSON, B. (1992) 'The construction of subjectivity and the paradox of resistance: reintegrating feminist anthropology and psychology', *Signs: Journal of Women in Culture and Society*, **18**, 1, pp. 44–73.

MALEK, M. (1993) *Passing the Buck: Institutional Responses to Controlling Children with Difficult Behaviour*, London, The Children's Society.

MAMA, A.(1995) *Beyond the Masks: Race, Gender and Subjectivity*, London, Routledge.

MAPSTONE, E. and DAVEY, G. (1990) 'Foreword: on being at a disadvantage', *The Psychologist: Bulletin of the British Psychological Society*, **13**, p. 387.

MARCHBANK, J. (1994) 'Non-decision-making . . . a management guide to keeping women's interest issues off the political agenda', in GRIFFIN, G., HESTER, M., RAI. S. and ROSENEIL, S. (Eds) *Stirring It: Challenges for Feminism*, London, Taylor & Francis.

MARCUSE, H. (1968) *One Dimensional Man: The Ideology of Industrial Society*, London, Sphere Books.

MARKS, D., BURMAN, E., BURMAN, L. and PARKER, I. (1995) 'Collaborative research into education case conferences', *Educational Psychology in Practice*, **11**, 1, pp. 41–9.

MARSHALL, A. (1994) 'Sensous sapphires: a study of the social construction of black female sexuality', in MAYNARD, M. and PURVIS, J. (Eds) *Researching Women's Lives from a Feminist Perspective*, London, Taylor & Francis.

MARSHALL, H. (1991) 'The social construction of motherhood: an analysis of childcare and parenting manuals', in PHOENIX, A., WOOLLETT, A. and LLOYD, E. (Eds) *Motherhood: Meanings, Practices and Ideologies*, London, Sage.

MARSHALL, R. (1988) 'The role of ideology in the individualisation of distress', *The Psychologist: Bulletin of the British Psychological Society*, **2**, pp. 67–9.

MARTIN, L. H., GUTMAN, H. and HUTTON, P. H. (Eds) (1988) *Technologies of the Self: A Seminar with Michel Foucault*, London, Tavistock Publications.

MARTIN, R. (1988) 'Truth, power, self: an interview with Michel Foucault', in MARTIN, L., GUTMAN, H. and HUTTON, P. (Eds) *Technologies of the Self*, London, Tavistock Publications.

MARX, K. (orig. 1844) 'The German ideology', in McLELLAN, D. (Ed. 1977) *Karl Marx: Selected Writings*, Oxford, Oxford University Press.

MARX, K. (orig. 1849) 'Wage labour and capital', in McLELLAN, D. (Ed. 1977) *Karl Marx: Selected Writings*, Oxford, Oxford University Press.

MARX, K. (orig. 1857) 'Grundrisse', in McLELLAN, D. (Ed. 1977) *Karl Marx: Selected Writings*, Oxford, Oxford University Press.

MICHAEL, M. (1994) 'The power-persuasion-identity nexus: anarchism and actor networks', *Anarchist Studies*, **2**, 1, pp. 25–42.

MILLER, P. (1987) *Domination and Power*, London, RKP.

MILLER, P. and ROSE, N. (Eds) (1986) *The Power of Psychiatry*, Cambridge, Polity Press.

MILLS, S. (Ed.) (1994) *Gendering the Reader*, Hemel Hempstead, Harvester Wheatsheaf.

References

MITCHELL, J. (1974) *Psychoanalysis and Feminism*, Harmondsworth, Pelican Books.

MMD/MAS update (1993) *Ethnic Minority Staff in the NHS: A Programme for Action*, update 12/93, held at North Manchester Health Authority.

MONEY, J. (1955) 'Hermaphroditism, gender and precocity in hyperadrenocorticism: psychologic findings', *Bulletin Johns Hopkins Hospital*, **96**, pp. 253–64.

NADIRSHAW, Z. (1993) 'Therapeutic practice in multiracial Britain', *Transcultural Psychiatry Society (UK) Bulletin*, **1**, pp. 1–4.

NAIRN, K. (1982) *Women and Depression*, London, The Women's Press.

NATIONAL HEALTH SERVICE TASK FORCE (1994a) *Black Mental Health: A Dialogue for Change*, London, Department of Health.

NATIONAL HEALTH SERVICE TASK FORCE (1994b) *Time for Action Now – Regional Race Programme: Greater Manchester Seminar*, London, Department of Health.

NEWSON, J. and NEWSON, E. (1974) 'Cultural aspects of childrearing in the English-speaking world', in RICHARDS, M. P. M. (Ed.) *The Integration of a Child into a Social World*, Cambridge, Cambridge University Press.

NICOLSON, P. (1992) 'Gender issues in the organisation of clinical psychology', in USSHER, J. and NICOLSON, P. (Eds) *Gender Issues in Clinical Psychology*, London, Routledge.

O'CONNOR, N. and RYAN, J. (1993) *Wild Desires and Mistaken Identities*, London, Virago.

O'HAGAN, K. and DILLENBURGER, K. (1995) *The Abuse of Women in Childcare Work*, Buckingham, Open University Press.

O'KEEFFE, D. (1994) 'Debunking the truancy myths', *The Guardian*, 4 January.

OLIVER, P. (1991) 'What do girls know anyway?: rationality, gender and social control', *Feminism and Psychology*, **1**, pp. 339–60.

ORBACH, S. (1978) *Fat is a Feminist Issue*, London, Paddington Press.

ORBACH, S. (1986) *Hunger Strike*, London, Faber & Faber.

OWUSU-BEMPAH and HOWITT, D. (1994) 'Racism and the psychological textbook', *The Psychologist: Bulletin of the British Psychological Society*, **7**, pp. 163–6.

PADEL, U. and STEVENSON, P. (1988) (Eds) *Insiders: Women's Experience of Prison*, London, Virago.

PARFREY, V. (1993) 'Excluding: failed children or systems failure?', Division of Educational and Child Psychology annual course, BPS, 5–8 January.

PARKER, I. (1989) *The Crisis in Modern Social Psychology and How to End It*, London, Routledge.

PARKER, I. (1992) *Discourse Dynamics: Critical Analysis for Social and Individual Psychology*, London, Routledge.

PARKER, I. (1995) 'Qualitative research II: resources', unpublished ms.

PARKER, I. (1996) 'Psychology, science fiction and postmodern space', *South African Journal of Psychology*, **26**, 3.

PARKER, I., GEORGACA, E., HARPER, D., McLAUGHLIN, T. and STOWELL SMITH, M. (1995) *Deconstructing Psychopathology*, London, Sage.

PARKER, I. and SHOTTER, J. (Eds) (1990) *Deconstructing Social Psychology*, London, Routledge.

PARMAR, P. (1988) 'Gender race and power: the challenge to youth work practice', in COHEN, P. and BAINS, H. (Eds) *Multi-Racist Britain*, Basingstoke, Macmillan.

PARMENTER, J. (1994) *Looking After Baby: Yesterday, Today ... Tomorrow, Trends in Infant Care Practice, Bristol 1951–1991*, Bristol, Redcliffe.

PARTON, N. (1991) *Governing the Family*, Basingstoke, Macmillan.

PHOENIX, A. (1987) 'Theories of gender and black families', in WEINER, G. and ARNOT, M. (Eds) *Gender Under Scrutiny: New Inquiries in Education*, Buckingham, Open University Press.

PHOENIX, A., WOOLLETT, A. and LLOYD, E. (Eds) (1991) *Motherhood: Meanings, Practices and Ideologies*, London, Sage.

PILGRIM, D. and TREACHER, A. (1991) *Clinical Psychology Observed*, London, Routledge.

POOVEY, M. (1988) 'Feminism and deconstruction', *Feminist Studies*, **14**, 1, pp. 51–65.

POTIER, M. (1993) 'Giving evidence: women's lives in Ashworth maximum security psychiatric hospital', *Feminism and Psychology*, **3**, 3, pp. 335–47.

PRIBOR, E. F. and DINWIDDIE, S. H. (1992) 'Psychiatric correlates of incest in childhood', *American Journal of Psychiatry*, **156**, pp. 52–6.

PROBYN, E. (1990) 'Travels in the postmodern: making sense of the local', in NICHOLSON, L. (Ed.) *Feminism/Postmodernism*, New York, Routledge.

PRU and JENNIFER (1994) 'WISH update', *WISH Newsletter*, 2, summer, London, WISH.

RACK, P. (1982) *Race, Culture and Mental Disorder*, London, Tavistock Publications.

RAMAZANOGLU, C. (1989) *Feminism and the Contradictions of Oppression*, London, Routledge.

RAMAZANOGLU, C. (Ed.) (1992) *Up Against Foucault: Explorations of Some Tensions Between Foucault and Feminism*, London, Routledge.

RATNA, L. and WHEELER, M. (1994) 'Race and gender issues in adult psychiatry', in BURCK, C. and SPEED, B. (Eds) *Gender, Power and Relationships*, London, Routledge.

RAYMOND, J. (1979) *The Transsexual Empire: The Making of the She-Male*, Boston, MA, Beacon.

REASON, P. and ROWAN, J. (Eds) (1981) *Human Inquiry: a Sourcebook of New Paradigm Research*, Chichester, John Wiley.

REED, J. (chair) (1994) *Report of the Working Party on High Security and Related Psychiatric Provision*, London, Department of Health.

REESE, H. W. and OVERTON, W. F. (1970) 'Models of development and theories of development', in GOULET, L. R. and BALTES, P. B. (Eds) *Life-span Developmental Psychology, Research and Theory*, New York, Academic Press.

REICHER, S. and PARKER, I. (1993) 'Psychology politics resistance – the birth of a new organization', *Journal of Community and Applied Social Psychology*, **3**, pp. 77–80.

RIDLEY, C. (1995) *Overcoming Unintentional Racism in Counseling and Therapy*, Beverly Hills, CA, Sage.

RILEY, D. (1983) *War in the Nursery: Theories of the Child and Mother*, London, Virago.

RIVIERE, J. (1929) 'Womanliness as a masquerade', reprinted in BURGIN, V., DONALD, J. and KAPLAN, C. (Eds) *Formations of Fantasy*, London, Methuen.

ROBINSON, M. (1993) *Spanning Communities of Practice, COMIC working document*, Esprit Basic Research Project 6225, 1st draft, January.

ROGERS, A., PILGRIM, D. and LACEY, R. (1993) *Experiencing Psychiatry: Users' Views of Services*, London, Macmillan/MIND.

ROSE, N. (1985) *The Psychological Complex*, London, Routledge & Kegan Paul.

ROSE, N. (1989) *Governing the Soul: The Shaping of the Private Self*, London, Routledge.

ROSE, N. and MILLER, P. (1992) 'Political power beyond the state: problematics of government', *British Journal of Sociology*, **43**, 2, June.

ROSE, S., LEWONTIN, R. and KAMIN, L. (1984) *Not in our Genes: Biology, Ideology and Human Nature*, Harmondsworth, Penguin Books.

ROTH, T. and LEIPER, R. (1995) 'Selecting for clinical training', *The Psychologist: Bulletin of the British Psychological Society*, **8**, pp. 25–8.

ROTMAN, B. (1980) *Piaget: Psychologist of the Real*, Brighton, Harvester.

ROWE, D. (1984) *The Experience of Depression*, Chichester, John Wiley.

ROWE, K. K. (1990) 'Roseanne: unruly woman as domestic goddess', *Screen*, **31**, 4, winter, pp. 408–19.

RUSHTON, A. (1995) 'Get them young! The effects of early intervention on children's social behaviour', in FARRELL, P. *Emotional and Behavioural Difficulties: Strategies for Assessment and Intervention*, London, Falmer Press.

RUSSELL, D. (1995) *Women, madness and medicine*, Cambridge, Polity Press.

RYAN, J. (1983) *Feminism and Therapy*, London, Polytechnic of North London.

SASHIDHARAN, S. and FRANCIS, E. (1993) 'Epidemiology, ethnicity and schizophrenia', in AHMAD, W. (Ed.) *'Race' and Health in Contemporary Britain*, Buckingham, Open University Press.

SAWICKI, J. (1991) *Disciplining Foucault: Feminism, Power and the Body*, London, Routledge.

SAYAL, A. (1990) 'Black women and mental health', *The Psychologist: Bulletin of the British Psychological Society*, **3**, pp. 24–7.

SCARRE, G. (Ed.) (1989) *Children, Parents and Politics*, Cambridge, Cambridge University Press.

SCHILLING, K. M. and FUEHRER, A. (1993) 'The politics of women's self-help books', *Feminism and Psychology*, **3**, 3, pp. 418–22.

SCOTT, S. and PAYNE, T. (1984) 'Underneath we're all lovable', *Trouble and Strife*, **3**, Summer, pp. 21–4.

SCULL, A. (1979) *Museums of Madness: The Social Organisation of Insanity in Nineteenth Century England*, London, Allen Lane.

SECRETARY OF STATE (1989) *White Paper: Working for Patients*, London, HMSO.

SHAPIRO, J. (1991) 'Transsexualism: reflections on the persistence of gender and the mutability of sex', in EPSTEIN, J. and STRAUB, K. (Eds) *Body Guards: The Cultural Politics of Gender Ambiguity*, New York, Routledge.

SHEPPERD, M. (1990) *Mental Health: the Role of the Approved Social Worker*, Joint Unit for Social Services Research, University of Sheffield/Community Care.

SHOWALTER, E. (1985) *The Female Malady: Women, Madness and English Culture, 1830–1980*, London, Virago.

SINASON, V. (1992) Mental Health and the Human Condition. London, Free Association Books.

SINGER, E. (1992) *Child-care and the Psychology of Development*, London, Routledge.

SINGLETON, V. and MICHAEL, M. (1993) 'Actor-networks and ambivalence: General Practitioners in the cervical screening programme', *Social Studies of Science*, **23**, pp. 227–64.

SMART, C. (1989) 'Power and the politics of child custody', in *Child Custody and the Politics of Gender*, London, Routledge.

SMITH, A. (orig. 1776) in SKINNER, A. (Ed. 1970) *The Wealth of Nations*, Harmondworth, Penguin Books.

SMITH, D. (1990) *Texts, Facts, and Femininity: Exploring the Relations of Ruling*, London, Routledge.

SMITH, H, (1991) 'Caring for everyone? the implications for women of the changes in community care services', *Feminism and Psychology*, **1**, pp. 279–92.

SPELMAN, E. V. (1988) *Inessential Woman: Problems of Exclusion in Feminist Thought*, London, The Women's Press.

SPENDER, D. (1980) *Man Made Language*, London, Routledge & Kegan Paul.

SPENDER, D. (1994) '1. Women and madness: a justifiable response', *Feminism and Psychology*, **4**, 2, pp. 280–3.

SPIVAK, G. C. (1988) *In Other Worlds: Essays in Cultural Politics*, New York, Routledge.

References

SPIVAK, G. C. (1989) 'Can the subaltern speak?', in NELSON, C. and GROSSBERG, L. (Eds) *Marxism and the Interpretation of Culture*, Urbana, IL, University of Illinois Press.

SQUIRE, C. (1990) 'Crisis, what crisis? Discourses and narratives of the "social" in social psychology', in PARKER, I. and SHOTTER, J. (Eds) *Deconstructing Social Psychology*, London, Routledge.

STALLYBRASS, P. and WHITE, A. (1986) *The Politics and Poetics of Transgression*, London, Methuen.

STANLEY, L. and WISE, S. (1983) *Breaking Out*, London, Routledge.

STANLEY, L. and WISE, S. (1993) *Breaking Out Again*, New Edition, London, Routledge.

STAR, S. L. (1991) 'Power, technology and the phenomenology of standards: on being allergic to onions', in LAW, J. (Ed.) *Power, Technology and the Modern World*, Sociological Review Monograph, London, Routledge.

STAR, S. L. and GRIESEMER, J. (1989) 'Institutional ecology, "translations" and boundary objects: amateurs and professionals in Berkeley's Museum of Vertebrate Zoology, 1907–39', *Social Studies of Science*, **19**, pp. 387–420.

STEVENSON, P. (1990) 'Containment or cure?' paper presented at the inaugural WISH conference, London.

STOLLER, R. (1968) *Sex and Gender, Vol. I*, New York, Jason Aronson.

STOLLER, R. (1975) *Sex and Gender, Vol. II*, New York, Jason Aronson.

STOLOROW, R. D., BRANDCHAFT, B. and ATWOOD, G. E. (1992) 'Intersubjectivity in psychoanalytic treatment', in GREGORY HAMILTON, N. (Ed.) *From Inner Sources: New Directions in Object Relations Psychotherapy*, Northvale, NJ, Jason Aronson.

STONE, A. R. (1991) 'The "Empire" strikes back: a posttransexual manifesto', in STRAUB, K. and EPSTEIN, J. (Eds) *Body Guards: The Cultural Politics of Gender Ambiguity*, New York, Routledge.

STOPPARD, M. (1995) *Complete Baby and Child Care*, London, Dorling Kindersley.

TAVRIS, C (1993) 'The mismeasure of woman', *Feminism and Psychology*, **3**, pp. 149–68.

TERRIE, (1994) 'Stability and security', *WISH Newsletter*, 19, summer, London, WISH.

THOMAS, C., STONE, K., OSBORN, M., THOMAS, P. and FISHER, M. (1993) 'Psychiatric morbidity and compulsory admission among UK-born Europeans, Afro–Caribbeans and Asians in Central Manchester', *British Journal of Psychiatry*, **163**, pp. 91–9.

TICKNER, L. (1987) *The Spectacle of Women: Imagery of the Suffrage Campaign 1907–14*, London, Chatto & Windus.

TORKINGTON, P. (1991) *Black Health – A Political Issue: The Health and Race Project*, Liverpool, CARJ-LIHE.

TULLY, B. (1992) *Accounting for Transsexualism and Transhomosexuality*, London, Whiting & Birch.

UDALL, L. (1994) 'Paul Hewitt has only one wish . . . to have his breasts and his womb removed', *The People*, **16** January, pp. 24–5.

URWIN, C. (1985) 'Constructing motherhood: the persuasion of normal development', in WALKERDINE, V., URWIN, C. and STEEDMAN, C. (Eds) *Language, Gender and Childhood*, London, Routledge & Kegan Paul.

URWIN, C. and SHARLAND, E. (1992) 'From bodies to minds in childcare literature: advice to parents in inter-war Britain', in COOTER, R. (Ed.) *In the Name of the Child*, London, Routledge.

USSHER, J. (1991) *Women's Madness: Misogyny or Mental Illness?* London, Harvester Wheatsheaf.

VAN KREIKEN, R. (1991) 'The poverty of social control: explaining power in the historical sociology of the welfare state', *Sociological Review,* **391**, 1, pp. 1–26.

VAN MENS-VERHULST, SCHREURS, K. and WOERTMAN, L. (Eds) (1993) *Daughtering and Mothering: Female Subjectivity Reanalysed*, London, Routledge.

VARELA, J. (1994) 'Foucault y las feministas', in PHILIPP, R. R. and NEGRO, M. C. G. *As mulleres: los cambios sociales e economicos*, Santiago de Compostela, Universidad de Santiago de Compostela, Spain.

VINCENT, S. (1993) 'Lost boys: a question of gender', *The Guardian Weekend*, 16 October, pp. 4–9.

VOLOSHINOV, V. N. (1973[1929]) *Marxism and the Philosophy of Language*, New York, Seminar Press.

WALKERDINE, V. (1981) 'Sex, power and pedagogy', *Screen Education*, **38**, pp. 14–25.

WALKERDINE, V. (1984) 'Developmental psychology and child-centred pedagogy', in HENRIQUES, J. *et al. Changing the Subject: Psychology, Social Regulation and Subjectivity*, London, Methuen.

WALKERDINE, V. (1988) *The Mastery of Reason: Cognitive Development and the Production of Rationality*, London, Routledge.

WALKERDINE, V. (1990) *Schoolgirl Fictions*, London, Verso.

WALKERDINE, V. and LUCEY, H. (1989) *Democracy in the Kitchen: Regulating Mothers and Socialising Daughters*, London, Virago.

WALLACE, M. (1990) *Black Macho and the Myth of the Superwoman*, New York, Verso.

WARD, L. (1993) 'Race, equality and employment in the National Health Service', in AHMAD, W. (Ed.) *'Race' and Health in Contemporary Britain*, Buckingham, Open University Press.

WARE, V. (1992) *Beyond the Pale: White Women, Racism and History*, London, Verso.

WEBB-JOHNSON, A. (1991) *A Cry for Change: An Asian Perspective on Developing Quality Mental Health Care*, London, Confederation of Indian Organisations (UK).

WEEDON, C. (1987) *Feminist Practice and Poststructuralist Theory*, Oxford, Basil Blackwell.

WEST, C. and ZIMMERMAN, D. (1991) 'Doing gender', in LORBER, J. and FARRELL, S. (Eds) *The Social Construction of Gender*, Beverly Hills, CA, Sage.

WHEELER, E. (1994) 'Doing black mental health research: observations and experiences', in AFSHAR, H. and MAYNARD, M. (Eds) *The Dynamics of 'Race' and Gender*, London, Taylor & Francis.

WHITE, R., CARR, P. and LOWE, N. (1990) *A Guide to the Children Act 1989*, London, Butterworths.

WHITNEY, B. (1993) *The Children Act and Schools*, London, Kogan Page.

WICOMB, Z. (1994) 'Motherhood and the surrogate reader: race, gender and interpretation', in MILLS, S. (Ed.) *Gendering the Reader*, Hemel Hempstead, Harvester Wheatsheaf.

WILKINSON, S. (1988) 'The role of reflexivity in feminist psychology', *Women's Studies International Forum*, **11**, 5, pp. 493–502.

WILLIAMS, J. and WATSON, G. (1993) 'Mental health services that empower women: the challenge to clinical psychology', *Clinical Psychology Forum*, **64**, pp. 6–12.

WILLIAMS, R. (1976) *Keywords: A vocabulary of culture and society*, London, Fontana.

WINNICOTT, D. W. (1971) *Playing and Reality*, Harmondsworth, Penguin Books.

WINNICOTT, D. W. (1986) *Home Is Where We Start From: Essays by a Psychoanalyst*, Harmondsworth, Penguin Books.

WOLMARK, J. (1995) 'Cyborg bodies and problems of representation', in BURMAN, E., GORDO LÓPEZ, A. J., MACAULEY, W. R. and PARKER, I. (Eds) *Cyberpsychology: Conference, Interventions and Reflections*, Manchester Discourse Unit, Manchester Metropolitan University.

WONG, L. (1994) 'Di(s)-secting and dis(s)-closing whiteness: two tales about psychology', *Feminism and Psychology*, **4**, pp. 133–54.

WORELL, J. and REMER, P. (1992) *Feminist Perspectives in Therapy – An Empowerment Model for Women*, New York, John Wiley.

WORRALL, A. (1990) *Offending Women: Female Lawbreakers and the Criminal Justice System*, London, Routledge.

YEBOAH, S. (1988) *The Ideology of Racism*, London, HANSIB.

YONEYAMA, J. and MARKUSSEN, R. (1993) 'Situated in the great divide', in BOWKER, G., STAR, S. L. and TURNER, W. (Eds) *Invited Workshop: Social Science Research, Technical Systems, and Cooperative Work*, Paris, Dep. Sciences Humaines et Sociales, Cnrs, March.

YUVAL-DAVIS, N. (1992) 'Fundamentalism, multiculturalism and women in Britain', in DONALD, J. and RATTANSI, A. (Eds) *'Race', Culture and Difference*, London, Sage.

ZIZEK, S. (1989) *The Sublime Object of Ideology*, London, Verso.

ZUCKERMAN, M. and BRODY, N. (1988) 'Oysters, rabbits and people: a critique of "race differences in behaviour" by J. P. Rushton', *Journal of Personality and Individual Differences*, **9**, 6, pp. 1025–33.

Index

UNIVERSITY OF WOLVERHAMPTON
LEARNING RESOURCES